*Also by Gayle Olinekova:*
Go For It!

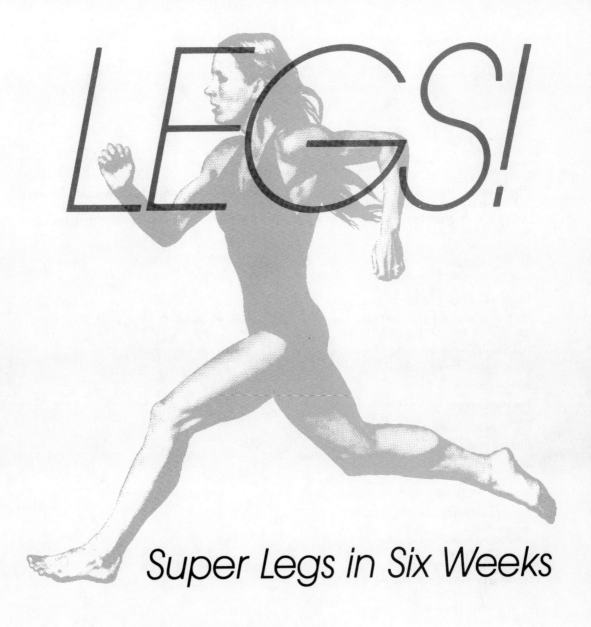

# LEGS!

*Super Legs in Six Weeks*

# BY GAYLE OLINEKOVA
## Photography Editor Michael Grandi

A FIRESIDE BOOK • PUBLISHED BY SIMON & SCHUSTER, INC. • NEW YORK

The instructions and advice in this book are in no way intended as a substitute for medical counseling. We advise anyone to consult with a doctor before beginning this or any regimen of exercise. The author and the publisher disclaim any liability or loss, personal or otherwise, resulting from the procedures in this book.

## Photo credits

Michael Grandi: 2, 4, 6, 8, 9, 44 right side, 48, 49, 72, 77, 78, 90, 93, 95, 96, 97, 98, 102, 103, 105, 106, 109, 112, 114, 115, 127, 128

Don Lauritzen: 20, 34, 35, 36, 37, 38, 39, 40, 41, 42, 43, 44 left side, 45, 46, 47, 51, 52, 53, 54, 55, 56, 57, 58, 117

Rick Semple: 50

Bill Heimanson: 111

Robert Riger: 5, 129

Richard Mackson: 120, 121

Manny Guttierrez: 122, 123

Copyright © 1983 by Gayle Olinekova
All rights reserved
including the right of reproduction
in whole or in part in any form
A Fireside Book
Published by Simon & Schuster, Inc.
Simon & Schuster Building
Rockefeller Center
1230 Avenue of the Americas
New York, New York 10020
FIRESIDE and colophon are registered trademarks of Simon & Schuster, Inc.
Designed by H. Roberts Design
Manufactured in the United States of America
Printed and bound by Halliday Lithograph
10  9  8  7  6  5  4  3  2

Library of Congress Cataloging in Publication Data

Olinekova, Gayle
  Legs: super legs in six weeks.

  "A Fireside book."
  1. Reducing exercises.  2. Exercise.  3. Leg.
4. Aerobic exercises.  5. Women—Nutrition.  I. Title.
RA781.6.O44  1983      613.7′1      82-618
ISBN 0-671-47241-0

# ACKNOWLEDGMENTS

Charts on pages 16–18 courtesy of Bermuda Inn.

The following books were helpful in preparing the manuscript:

*Materia Medica* by William Boericke, M.D.
*Back to Eden* by Jethro Kloss
*How to Get Well* by Paavo Airola, N.D., Ph.D.

Medical Consultants:

Dr. Jack Kahn, D.C.
Dr. Kenneth Rehm, D.P.M.

Typing: Edith Butler
Photographic Equipment: Irwyn Grief

And a special thanks to a special person—my editor, Angela Miller, who matches her erudite professionalism with kindness and an incandescent personality.

To my guardian angels,
who have been working overtime for years.

# CONTENTS

# LEGS!

# License to Succeed

### THIS IS TO CERTIFY THAT

_____

### IS HEREBY LICENSED TO

# succeed

### IN OWNING A PAIR OF

# super legs!

DATE _____ SIGNED _Gayle Olinekova_

# INTRODUCTION

*Only the belief that we have limitations holds us back.*

The ad campaign says it all. "Nothin' beats a great pair of legs." They're right—nothing does. Your legs account for more than *half* your body structure. The femur bones are also the largest bones of the body, and attached to them are the largest muscles.

Men and women all over the world have stopped me to ask the inevitable question, "Where did you get those legs?" And when *Sports Illustrated* gave me the title "The Greatest Legs to Ever Stride the Earth," telegrams and letters poured in from all over the world asking the same question.

Well, they didn't just come in the mail one day. My legs used to be skinny. And once they were just plain old *fat* legs. But from each sport I've been in—ocean rowing, speedskating, and cycling to sprinting, modern dance, and marathon running—and from each and every injury an athlete who competes as I do is almost destined to get, I've gleaned the secrets and supermethods of the Olympic athletes and star performers from all over the world.

You can develop your legs into great legs with these methods. I've used them, and they've certainly worked for me.

Interviewers often ask me what it's like to have "The Greatest Legs." There are so many answers.

The fact that people find my legs to be beautiful is an honor—one that really humbles me—and I appreciate that people find pleasure in the aesthetics of the way they look. But it's when I *do* something with them that they give *me* pleasure—and it's the physical activities that got them that way in the first place.

It feels terrific to have "the greatest legs." For instance, it means knowing the exhilaration of having my legs take me to the finish tape after running 26.2 miles to get there. It's being able to walk up the side of a mountain and not be tired, and then see a view from the top so magnificent you get goosebumps. And it's being able to dance all night long and never feel like your legs need to rest.

You see, sculpting a new shape for your legs is exciting and fulfilling, and it doesn't matter if you are rich or poor, tall or short, fat or skinny. There have been times in my life when I've been poorest, when I was living on a skateboard budget but, running down the street, my body was handling like a finely tuned Porsche.

Everyone can have better legs. Why shuffle through life, too tired to cope? Stride through with confidence. You can with the methods in this book.

Surprisingly, one of the first questions people usually ask when it comes to exercise is, "Will lifting weights and exercising cause a woman to lose her femininity?"

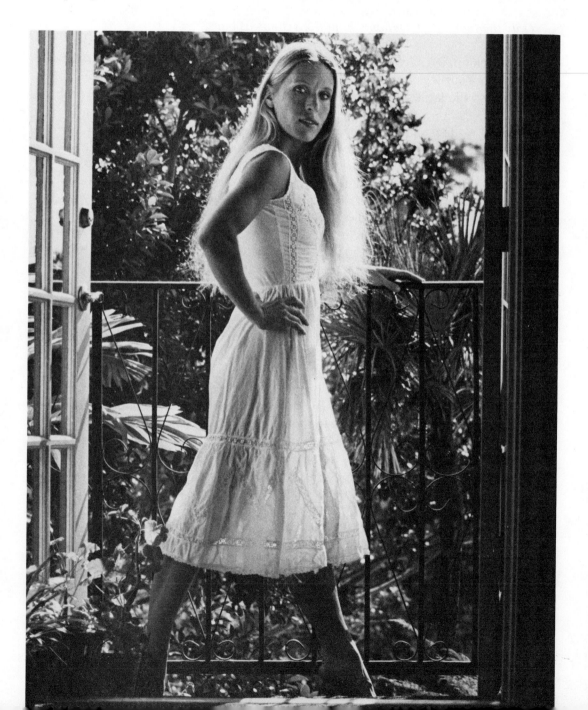

The only way for a woman to lose her femininity is on the operating table. As any dancer will tell you, grace and beautiful movement come from power. Think of a ballerina lifting her leg off the ground and straight up over her head. Looks beautiful. It takes an enormous amount of power and strength to achieve that beauty. Try it out for yourself.

Frankly, I'm more surprised that more people don't ask, "Does cellulite cause a woman to lose her femininity?" It certainly obscures the sinewy natural line of a woman's body.

If you have cellulite, don't despair. Even if you've had it so long it feels as though you were *born* with it, you *can* get rid of it. Thin thighs can be yours if you're willing to do something about it. I'll show you how.

Some women (and men) also suffer from another leg malady sometimes referred to unkindly as "toothpickitis"; that is, skinny legs. When you go to the beach, do you feel like you're sinking in the sand right up to your knees? This book is also for you. Shapely legs are always in style—and now you can learn how to sculpt yours into great legs.

But exercise is not the whole answer. I've seen some of the world's top women marathon runners with possibly the world's skinniest bodies *also* have cellulite on their legs from the knees up! Diet is a great factor here, and their legs would obviously look much worse if they didn't run a step, but more on food later in the diet section.

As you sit there now, holding this book in your hands, perhaps you're wondering in a small voice somewhere inside of you if this is all going to be worth it. Let's face it, you've got some energy output ahead of you. It's not easy to be in shape and have a great pair of legs. If it took no effort, then *everybody* would look terrific.

You can't decide if it's not worth going for until you do—and *then* count the cost. But when summer comes, and you slip into your new French-cut designer jeans or teenie bikini, think of how glad you'll be that you took the trouble to get super legs. You'll be spending the rest of your life inside that body of yours. Make it a classy place to live!

So congratulations on wanting just a little bit more out of life. Now turn the page and let's get to it!

## Why Six Weeks?

Living in Hollywood, I was accustomed to getting frantic calls from movie stars who had just been given the shooting schedule for their latest project. Usually they

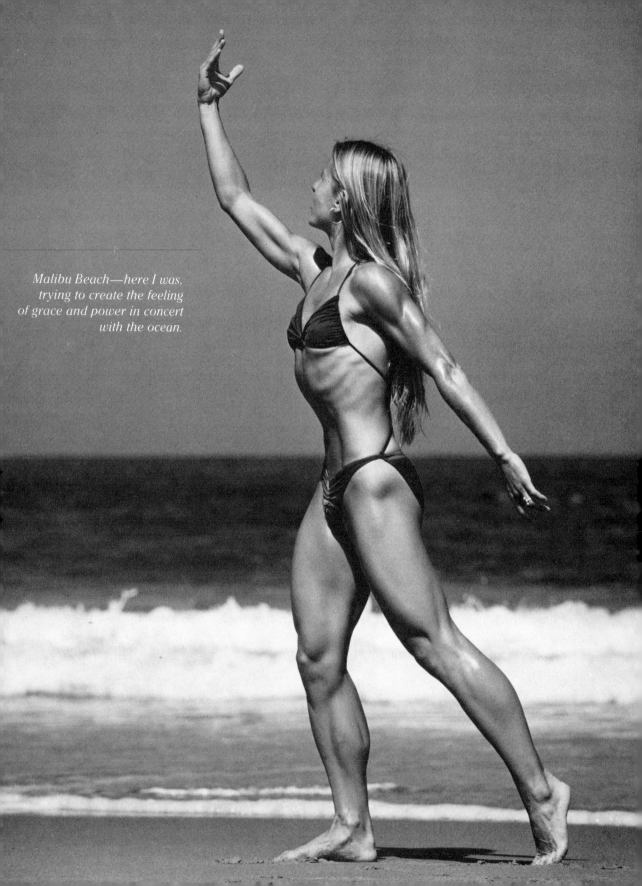

*Malibu Beach—here I was, trying to create the feeling of grace and power in concert with the ocean.*

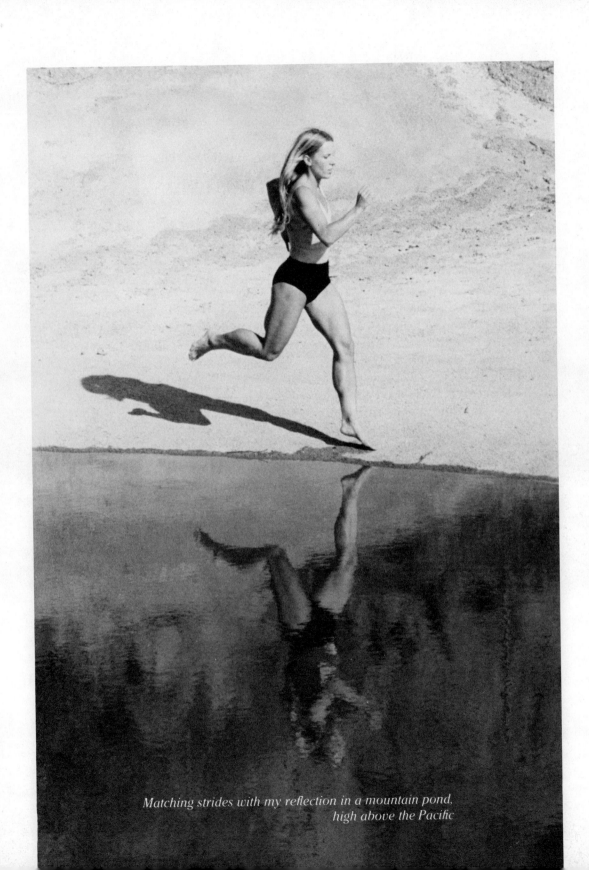

*Matching strides with my reflection in a mountain pond,
high above the Pacific*

had between four to six weeks to get ready for the part, and they had to get in shape *fast*. It *had* to be done, their director demanded!

As you may know, the camera unkindly adds ten to twenty pounds, automatically making you appear heavier than you actually are. So even the stars who have only let it slide a *little* bit still have to worry about that extra "camera weight."

Six weeks is plenty of time. Of course, it means *every single day* of that six weeks has to be devoted to the task at hand. Obviously, if it has been twenty-five years since you've done a spot of exercise, you're going to have to expect to work harder and keep doing it, but after six weeks you'll be amazed at the results.

The next six weeks are your "launching" weeks. It is important to follow each step carefully and exactly. No substitutions. Day by day you'll be getting stronger— developing new muscle tissue, firming up flab, tightening the skin, using up fat. Each facet of the program is designed to make you better every day. Enjoy it. If it works for the stars, it can work for you.

The next six weeks are only the beginning. You will soon discover that a new personal power is yours. You are a person who succeeds today in your fitness program, tomorrow in your job, the following day in whatever you wish for.

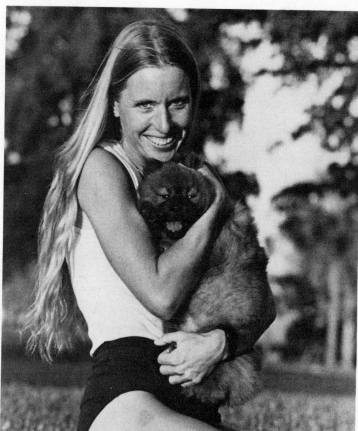

*Take Fido with you when you walk or run, but only if he's trained to stay with you.*

# CELLULITE

Fifty years ago, cellulite was quite uncommon, almost unknown on our continent. It is still unknown in cultures we call "primitive"—people in the sparse groups around the world who are still eating the diets established in traditions handed down by their ancestors through the centuries. This would seem to indicate that cellulite is not inherited—not something we are condemned to go through life with.

Look at old high-school yearbooks from the thirties and forties, or family snapshots from those times. Even though some people in the photos may have been overweight, they probably *didn't* have cellulite. Yet I've coached high-school track teams where some of the fourteen-year-old girls on the team had cellulite. Why?

Cellulite is *not* some mistake Nature made on us. It is an indication that somehow we have made more than a few mistakes in the way we treat ourselves. Actually, we could say this about most of our "civilized" ailments—from high blood pressure, hardening of the arteries, and varicose veins to hypoglycemia, hemorrhoids, and acne.

Cellulite, however, is not a disease, regardless of how destestable it may seem to us. It's not a real medical condition, or even a correct anatomical term! "Cellulitis" is the closest you'll find in your *Merck Manual* and that refers to secondary skin infections.

Cellulite is the lay person's term for that dimply, bumpy, fatty, and often hanging skin that seems to accumulate on the hips, thighs, and buttocks of great numbers of the female population. Men seem to be less afflicted by it due to the male hormone testosterone, although if they *do* have it, it's usually around their middle—from the belly button to the tailbone in a roll of fat. Estrogen, the hormone most prevalent in women, encourages the female body to store a layer of fat as a hedge to sustain future pregnancies.

Preservatives, artificial coloring and flavoring, refined carbohydrates (especially white bread and sugar), table salt, alcohol, and last but certainly not least, *hydrogenated fats* are some of the ingredients of the modern diet that experts are now shaking their fingers at.

Hydrogenated fats are those fats that stay solid at room temperature, i.e., margarine and vegetable shortening, and a host of oils used in foods ranging from chocolate bars and peanut butter to breakfast cereals and spaghetti sauce. These are thought to be the biggest culprits by Dr. Jack Kahn, the man who developed the science of Nutripathology–the nutrient-dosing approach to pathological disorders of the body. "The hydrogenated fat doesn't break down the way Nature intended after

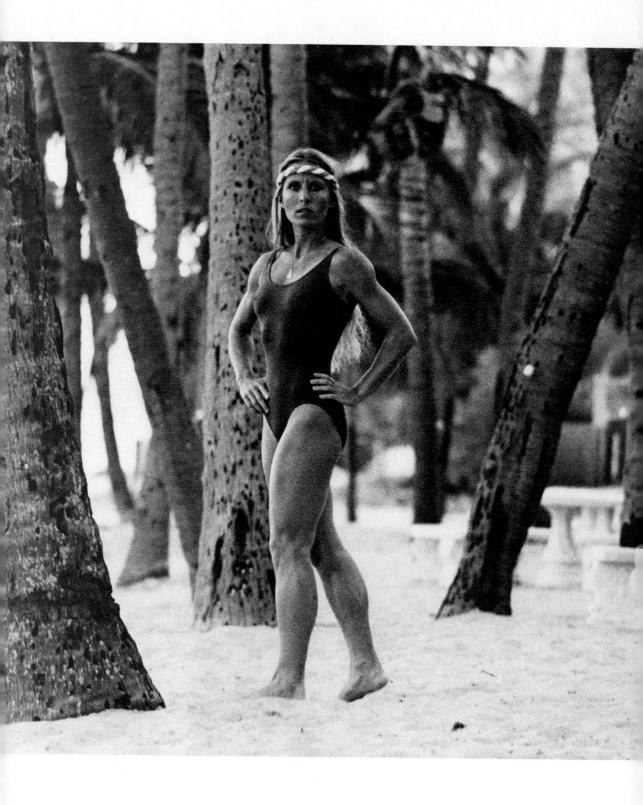

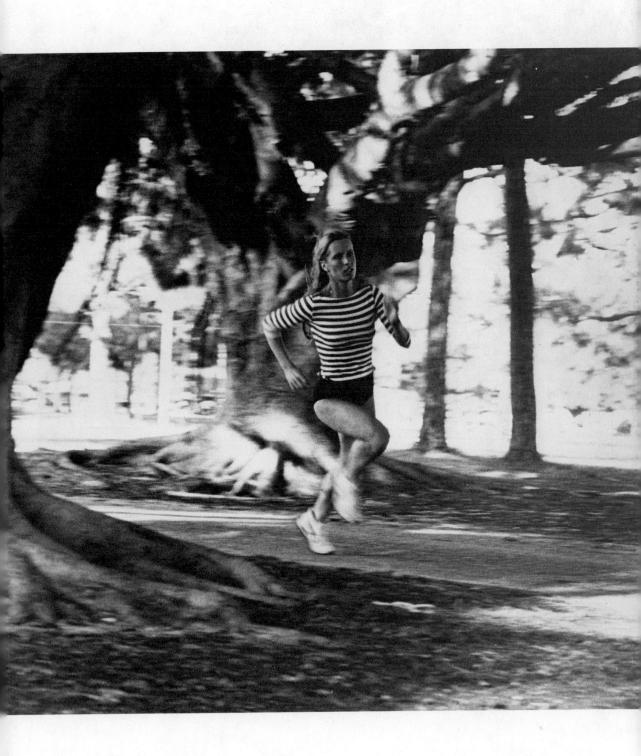

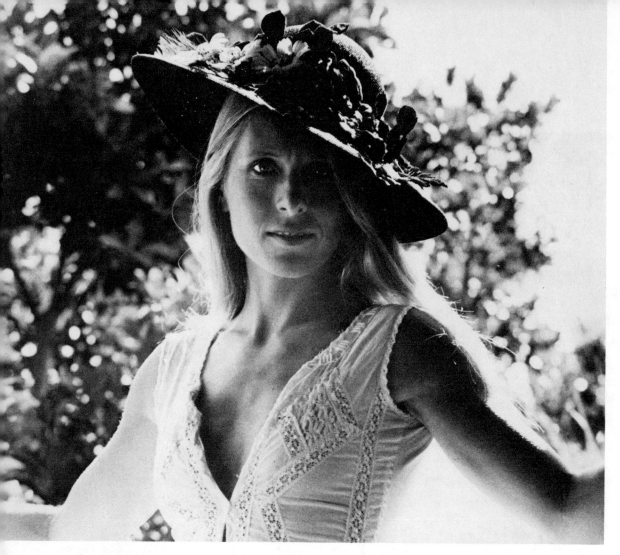

these tampered-with fats enter the body." He explains how, combined with lack of exercise, these incompletely broken-down fats must then be stored somehow as body fat.

Unattractively as fat on the body may have been stored in the past, at least it was laid down smoothly and behaved itself under the skin. Now it's not even plain old fat. It's *cellulite!* Maybe all those food additives and preservatives are serving another function these days, other than giving shelf life to the products. Perhaps they're preserving fat so that it hangs around longer in the form of saddlebags on our thighs and derrière!

Who needs it? Absolutely no one. You don't *have* to have it. Follow these guidelines and fight cellulite. It's a battle you must wage yourself, but the rewards are great.

Those super legs you were only able to *dream* about in the past can be yours for the rest of your life!

**Fight Cellulite** _____

1. Get plenty of exercise.

2. Cut out salt.

3. Cut down your fat intake—add no oils or fats to your food.*

4. Read labels. Do *not* buy or eat foods containing hydrogenated fats.

5. Add lecithin granules to your food (salads, sauces, etc.). It helps to emulsify dietary fat.

6. Garlic also helps to emulsify dietary fat. Press fresh garlic on salads. Add to soups and sauces for flavor. It's also famous as an aphrodisiac.

7. Avoid sitting—it impedes circulation. If your job calls for it, periodically flex all the muscles in your derrière and legs to keep blood circulating.

8. Give your legs a "facial." (See page 23.)

9. Avoid tight clothing that restricts circulation, i.e., tight jeans, girdles, garters.

10. Ensure your vitamin intake of E, C, and the minerals—especially calcium and magnesium.

11. Exercise, exercise, exercise! Good bets: swimming—do the kickboard exercises *religiously;* do the walk/run uphill workouts.

_____

# LOSING WEIGHT PAINLESSLY

When you're hungry, eat. When you're not hungry, don't eat. This is the key to eating less, which is the absolutely foolproof weight-loss technique.

Do you know how much you really do eat? Perhaps you don't even realize just how much it is. The best way to find out in a hurry is simply to write it down. Buy a small 49¢ notebook. Keep it with you 24 hours a day and write down every single thing that goes in your mouth. Take a bite out of your kid's brownie? Write it down.

_____

* See *The Pritikin Diet* if you need help here. (Nathan Pritikin, New York: Grosset & Dunlap, 1979.)

Eat seven almonds while you're looking in the refrigerator? Write it down. Don't cheat on this, because it's for your eyes only.

Do this writing down for three days. You'll be surprised when you see what you've actually eaten. Now you can understand yourself more. Then you can cut out the obvious bad stuff that you ate when you were depressed, bored, or whatever.

Writing down the list of food makes you accountable to yourself, and this is very important. This is *your* thing, *your* fitness program—something that no one can take away from you.

If you want to count calories, buy one of those pocket calorie counters and go to it. This will reveal even more to you about how good or bad your eating habits are.

## Natural Food: Where Did It Grow?

When you are eating junk food, you have to eat more calories than is necessary to be satisfied. Junk food is basically empty of nutrients, so your body's appetite control mechanism (called the appestat) does not signal satiation until a large number of calories and a great quantity of food has been consumed. Your appestat signals "more food" until there is a sufficient supply of food nutrients.

For instance, I've known people who could eat a whole loaf of white bread at one meal, but when they eat two slices of homemade dark rye bread, they're full. The difference here is possibly 1,500 calories for the white bread and 200 calories for the whole-grain rye bread.

Eat "real" foods when you're hungry. You should be able to answer "Where did it grow?" before you eat it. For example: apple. Where did it grow? That's easy: an apple tree. Here's another one: chocolate eclair. Where did it grow? Tough to answer that one—and if you can't answer it, don't eat it. Caramel candy—where did it grow? Are you getting the idea? Soon, your big surprise will be that you don't have to diet. You will be living the eating plan you need.

Eating whole foods will keep you slender and fit easily into your life if you can make this your motto.

**WHEN YOU'RE HUNGRY, EAT.**
**WHEN YOU'RE NOT HUNGRY, DON'T EAT.**

Respect these words, and you're well on your way to owning the body you always wanted. Bon appetit!

# CALORIE CHARTS AND EXERCISE CHARTS FOR CHEATERS

**EXERCISE AND CALORIES**

| Activity | Approximate Calories Used | | | |
|---|---|---|---|---|
| | **1hr** | **½ hr** | **¼ hr** | **5 mins** |
| Walking (slow, 2 mph) | 150 | 75 | 38 | 13 |
| Walking (medium, 3 mph) | 300 | 150 | 75 | 25 |
| Walking (fast, 5 mph) | 480 | 240 | 120 | 40 |
| Golf (with power cart) | 200 | 100 | 50 | 17 |
| Golf (carrying bag) | 360 | 180 | 90 | 30 |
| Typical housework | 300 | 150 | 75 | 25 |
| Scrubbing floors | 360 | 180 | 90 | 30 |
| Bowling | 300 | 150 | 75 | 25 |
| Bicycling (slow, 6 mph) | 300 | 150 | 75 | 25 |
| Bicycling (medium, 8 mph) | 400 | 200 | 100 | 33 |
| Bicycling (fast) | 600 | 300 | 150 | 50 |
| Tennis (doubles) | 360 | 180 | 90 | 30 |
| Tennis (singles) | 480 | 240 | 120 | 40 |
| Ice/Roller skating | 420 | 210 | 105 | 35 |
| Jogging (slow, 5 mph) | 600 | 300 | 150 | 50 |
| Running (medium, 6 mph) | 700 | 350 | 175 | 58 |
| Skiing (downhill) | 600 | 300 | 150 | 50 |
| Lawn mowing (power mower) | 250 | 125 | 63 | 21 |
| Lawn mowing (hand mower) | 300 | 150 | 75 | 25 |
| Swimming (medium) | 400 | 200 | 100 | 33 |

These figures are approximate and calculated for a 150-lb. person.

## EXERCISE CHART FOR CHEATERS

Figures are based on data for a 150-lb. person, so lighter or heavier people will use fewer or more calories accordingly. An athlete in excellent condition will also use fewer calories due to oxygen efficiency. Figures are approximate and are based on information from USDA food charts.

| Food | Weight 1 oz = approx. 30 grams | Calories | Walking | Bicycling | Swimming | Jogging |
|---|---|---|---|---|---|---|
| | gm | kcal | min | min | min | min |
| Asparagus, cooked, 4 spears ............................ | 60 | 10 | 2 | 2 | 1 | 1 |
| Angel food cake, 1 pc (¹⁄₁₂ of 10″ cake)..................... | 53 | 135 | 26 | 20 | 16 | 14 |
| Apple, raw, 1 med (2½″ diam)............................ | 150 | 87 | 17 | 13 | 10 | 9 |
| Almonds, dried, salted, 12–15 nuts..................... | 15 | 93 | 18 | 14 | 11 | 9 |
| Almond bar, chocolate, 1 bar (1¼ oz) .................... | 38 | 310 | 60 | 46 | 36 | 31 |
| Blue Cheese (Roquefort) dressing ....................... | 14 | 70 | 14 | 10 | 8 | 7 |
| Bacon, lettuce, tomato sandwich—1 white toasted........... | 148 | 282 | 54 | 42 | 34 | 28 |
| Bologna with mayonnaise, sandwich 1 slice; tsp ............... | 68 | 220 | 42 | 33 | 26 | 22 |
| Beer, 8 oz glass .................................... | 240 | 115 | 22 | 18 | 14 | 12 |
| Bread (fresh & toasted) white, rye, whole wheat, Italian, French), 1 slice..................................... | 23 | 60 | 12 | 9 | 7 | 6 |
| Bread, buttered, 1 slice, 1 pat ........................... | 28 | 96 | 18 | 15 | 11 | 10 |
| Biscuit, honey, 2″ diam; 1 pat; 1 tsp ....................... | 40 | 164 | 32 | 25 | 19 | 16 |
| Bacon, crisp fried, 2 strips (20 strips/lb) ................... | 15 | 90 | 17 | 14 | 11 | 9 |
| Banana split ....................................... | 300 | 594 | 114 | 89 | 71 | 59 |
| Banana, 1 med ..................................... | 150 | 127 | 24 | 19 | 15 | 13 |
| Beef TV dinner..................................... | 310 | 350 | 67 | 52 | 42 | 35 |
| Broccoli, 1 stalk (5½″) ............................... | 100 | 32 | 6 | 5 | 4 | 3 |
| Cauliflower, cooked, drained, ⅛ cup ..................... | 105 | 31 | 6 | 5 | 4 | 3 |
| Corn, sweet, canned, ½ cup............................ | 128 | 85 | 16 | 13 | 10 | 9 |
| Chicken TV dinner, fried .............................. | 310 | 542 | 104 | 81 | 65 | 54 |
| Chicken noodle soup ................................. | 240 | 62 | 12 | 10 | 7 | 6 |
| Caramel, 1 oz....................................... | 30 | 118 | 23 | 18 | 14 | 12 |
| Chocolate milk, teacup (6½ oz) ......................... | 200 | 210 | 40 | 32 | 25 | 21 |
| Coca-Cola, 8 oz glass ................................ | 240 | 105 | 20 | 16 | 12 | 11 |
| Coffee & sugar, 1 cup; 1 tsp............................ | 200 | 30 | 6 | 5 | 4 | 3 |

| Food | Weight 1 oz = approx. 30 grams | Calories | Walking | Bicycling | Swimming | Jogging |
|---|---|---|---|---|---|---|
| | gm | kcal | min | min | min | min |
| Chili con carne, no beans, 1 cup | 250 | 334 | 64 | 50 | 40 | 33 |
| Chicken breast, broiled, ½ breast (no bone) | 72 | 105 | 20 | 16 | 13 | 11 |
| Chicken breast, fried, ½ breast (no bone) | 76 | 155 | 29 | 23 | 19 | 16 |
| Cupcake with icing, 1 (2½" diam) | 36 | 130 | 25 | 20 | 16 | 13 |
| Cottage cheese, 1 round tbs | 30 | 30 | 6 | 4 | 4 | 3 |
| Cheese, American, 1 slice (1 oz) | 30 | 112 | 22 | 17 | 13 | 11 |
| Cheese, toasted sandwich | 85 | 286 | 55 | 43 | 34 | 29 |
| Cheeseburger | 180 | 462 | 89 | 69 | 55 | 46 |
| Doughnut, 1 average | 32 | 125 | 24 | 19 | 15 | 13 |
| Egg, fried or scrambled, 1 med; 1 tsp oil | 53 | 108 | 21 | 16 | 13 | 11 |
| Fruit cocktail, ½ cup, water pack | 100 | 37 | 7 | 6 | 4 | 4 |
| French dressing | 14 | 57 | 11 | 9 | 7 | 6 |
| Frankfurter (1 frank 8/lb pkg) | 56 | 170 | 32 | 26 | 20 | 17 |
| Grapefruit juice, ½ glass (4 oz) | 120 | 47 | 9 | 7 | 6 | 5 |
| Hamburger, cooked 1 patty (3" diam x 1") | 85 | 224 | 43 | 34 | 27 | 22 |
| Hamburger | 150 | 350 | 57 | 52 | 42 | 35 |
| Hot dog with ketchup | 110 | 258 | 50 | 39 | 31 | 26 |
| Italian dressing | 14 | 100 | 19 | 15 | 12 | 10 |
| Ice cream—1 scoop | 60 | 115 | 22 | 17 | 14 | 12 |
| Ice cream bar, choc. coated, 1 bar | 60 | 195 | 37 | 30 | 23 | 20 |
| Lettuce, iceberg, ⅛ head (4¾" diam) | 55 | 10 | 2 | 2 | 1 | 1 |
| Low calorie dressing | 14 | 15 | 3 | 2 | 2 | 1 |
| Lobster, boiled with butter; 2 tbs butter | 334 | 308 | 59 | 46 | 37 | 31 |
| Mayonnaise | 14 | 100 | 19 | 15 | 12 | 10 |
| Milk, whole, 8 oz glass | 240 | 160 | 31 | 25 | 19 | 16 |
| Martini, cocktail, 3½ oz | 100 | 140 | 27 | 22 | 16 | 14 |
| Meatloaf TV dinner | 310 | 370 | 71 | 56 | 44 | 37 |

| Food | Weight 1 oz = approx. 30 grams | Calories | Walking | Bicycling | Swimming | Jogging |
|------|------|------|------|------|------|------|
| | gm | kcal | min | min | min | min |
| Mushrooms, fried, 4 med ................................. | 70 | 78 | 15 | 12 | 9 | 8 |
| Melba toast, unsalted, 1 thin slice ......................... | 4 | 15 | 3 | 2 | 2 | 2 |
| Milk, buttermilk, 8 oz glass ............................. | 240 | 88 | 17 | 13 | 10 | 9 |
| Orange, raw, 1 med (3″ diam) ........................... | 150 | 73 | 14 | 11 | 9 | 7 |
| Orange juice, ½ glass (4 oz) ............................ | 120 | 54 | 10 | 8 | 6 | 5 |
| Pork chops, lean, 2 chops (3 oz cooked) ................... | 90 | 260 | 49 | 39 | 31 | 26 |
| Peanuts, roasted, 6–8 nuts............................. | 15 | 86 | 17 | 13 | 10 | 9 |
| Peanuts, dry roasted, 8–10 nuts ........................ | 16 | 80 | 15 | 12 | 10 | 8 |
| Pretzels, 3 ring, 4 (148/lb) ............................. | 12 | 48 | 9 | 7 | 6 | 5 |
| Popsicle ............................................. | 95 | 70 | 4 | 10 | 8 | 7 |
| Pancake, 4″ diam........................................ | 45 | 105 | 20 | 16 | 12 | 11 |
| Pancake & syrup, 4″ diam; 2 tbs ......................... | 85 | 204 | 39 | 31 | 24 | 20 |
| Peach with cottage cheese; 2 med halves; 2 tbs cheese ........ | 156 | 105 | 20 | 16 | 13 | 10 |
| Potato salad, ½ cup .................................... | 100 | 99 | 19 | 15 | 12 | 10 |
| Peanut butter and jelly; 1 rounded tbs; 1 level tbs.............. | 86 | 290 | 55 | 45 | 35 | 29 |
| Pizza, sausage, ⅛ of 14″ dia pie........................... | 75 | 195 | 38 | 29 | 23 | 20 |
| Peas, green, cooked, ½ cup ............................. | 80 | 58 | 11 | 9 | 7 | 6 |
| Potato, baked with butter, 1 med; 2 pats ..................... | 110 | 160 | 31 | 24 | 19 | 16 |
| Raisins, dried; 1 tbs.................................... | 10 | 30 | 6 | 4 | 4 | 3 |
| Sunflower seeds, 30–40 nuts ............................. | 15 | 84 | 16 | 13 | 10 | 8 |
| Shrimp, French fried, 3½ oz. ............................ | 100 | 225 | 43 | 34 | 27 | 23 |
| Tomato soup .......................................... | 245 | 90 | 17 | 14 | 11 | 9 |
| Turkey, roasted, 2 slices; (3″ x 3½″) ...................... | 80 | 160 | 31 | 24 | 19 | 16 |
| Turkey, roasted with gravy, 2 slices; 2 tbs.................. | 115 | 240 | 46 | 36 | 29 | 24 |
| Tomato, tuna salad, 1 med; 2 tbs ........................ | 180 | 100 | 19 | 15 | 12 | 10 |
| T-bone steak, broiled, 3 oz cooked........................ | 90 | 175 | 33 | 26 | 21 | 18 |
| Waffle, plain, 5½″ diam. ................................ | 120 | 345 | 66 | 52 | 41 | 35 |
| Watermelon, 1 wedge (4″ x 8″) ........................... | 10 | 30 | 6 | 4 | 4 | 3 |

# WANT TO BE A SENSATION IN YOUR TEENIE BIKINI?

There are a few things you'll just *have* to give up!

- **SALT**—Because water retention in the body is Enemy # 1 for cellulite fighters.

- **FRYING**—Broil, bake, or roast.

- **FRENCH FRIES**—Puberty *is* over.

- **FAD DIETS**—They last only as long as the fad.

- **BOOZE**—Empty calories. If you must, have a wine spritzer (sparkling water and wine).

- **RED MEAT EVERY DAY**—Even the leanest steak can be 40 percent fat. Stick to chicken (skin removed), if you must eat meat, and fish. Investigate tofu as a protein source.

- **THOSE LATE-NIGHT SNACKS**—Remember the old adage: "Reach for your mate instead of your plate."

- **STAND-UP MEALS IN FRONT OF THE REFRIGERATOR**—Just because you eat it really fast, and nobody sees you, doesn't mean it doesn't count!

# SKINNY LEGS

Many people suffer from a malady unkindly referred to as "toothpickitis"—or skinny legs. With legs that are very thin, it's not really so much a matter of the leg measurements but the leg *shape* that counts.

Often the leg will continue down from the knee and seem to be an absolutely straight stalk, with no curves on it. This condition (or lack of condition) in the lower leg is enough to cause many women to wear long skirts and pants, and cause many men to avoid wearing shorts at all costs.

If this is *your* case, don't despair. The voluptuous curves of nicely developed calves *can* be yours. Pay particular attention to the lower leg and foot exercises on pages 34–47. Selecting running, walking, or cycling as your activity would also be a good choice for you—as would jumping rope. Walking barefoot in the soft sand at the beach, or in exercise sandals around the house is another good way for you to develop curves in your legs.

In the winter, try walking in freshly fallen snow—off the beaten track. Aerobic dancing is yet another way to super legs.

You are actually at an advantage having extremely thin legs. Other people have to lose fat and cellulite off their legs *first,* and *then* see their legs taking shape. You will see changes right away on your legs after you start working on them.

Soon, you'll be walking with more spring in your step, and looking to raise your hemlines, too. Skinny legs? Not anymore!

## WHAT CAUSES VARICOSE VEINS?

Inside the blood vessels that branch throughout the legs, there are innumerable tiny valves that keep the blood circulating. When pressure is put on these veins, such as with heart problems, pregnancy, obesity, tight jeans or garters, for instance, then the valves overload and stop working. The smaller surface veins are then called into action. As they were not made to handle the extra work, they stretch out and become bulging, ropy, blue-colored veins. These are varicose veins.

Improper diet and lack of certain vitamins are other causes, the chief one being lack of exercise and long periods of standing without movement. Salespeople, factory workers, and cashiers—please tune in here. Constipation is another main cause of varicose veins, as straining at the toilet can stretch the veins—hemorrhoids technically being varicose veins of the anus.

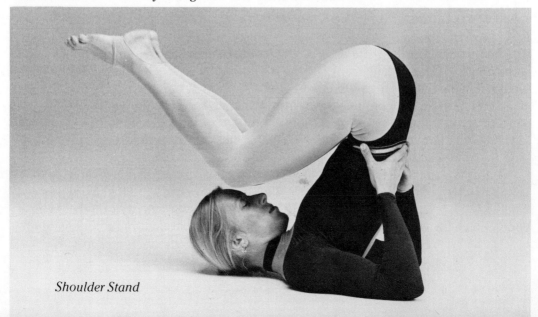

*Shoulder Stand*

## Very Good Tips for Varicose Veins

- Cut out salt.

- Exercise—an exercise bicycle is ideal (see page 85). Even in advanced stages, exercise will help.

- Elevate legs at every chance, especially while sleeping. This helps reduce swelling and drain blood.

- Shoulder Stand. This revives legs and is also great for your face—it helps prevent wrinkles.

- Walk in water.

- Increase vitamins E and C. Believe it or not, I had varicose veins at seventeen years of age. I found that increasing my vitamin E to 400 units twice a day, and vitamin C bioflavinoids to 3,000 milligrams per day, plus a good multimineral, worked. I no longer have even so much as a mark on my legs now (and I don't expect any).

- Check with your physician if you have emphysema or a heart condition.

- Eat a diet big in roughage. Eat plenty of fruit, salads, and whole grains, including bran.

- Herbs. Teas of sassafras, sweet marjoram, or marigold are old folk remedies. (See page 27 for Compress for Varicose Veins.)

*Note:* Of course, smoking is out of the question. Hasn't everyone stopped yet?

## Very Close Veins *(Spider Telangiectasia)*

These are the thin spidery webs of tiny little veins which seem to be very close to the surface of the skin. They are one of the signs of capillary fragility, a medical term which denotes the fragile condition of the miniature blood vessels of the body. They are not varicose veins, but if you follow the "Very Good Tips for Varicose Veins," especially watching your vitamin intake, you'll be preventing further developments.

Discoloration can sometimes be removed by a solution of equal parts of glycerine and cayenne pepper. *Caution: Do not use near eyes or mucous membranes!*

# GROOMING TIPS FOR SUPER LEGS

• Perfume behind your knees or on an ankle allows the scent to diffuse more effectively than the usual places.

• Wearing knee socks or shorter hemlines? Try some blush on your knees. It was considered very racy in the Roaring Twenties.

• Keep the body in balance with clothes—high-cut or "French-cut" legs on your leotard or swimsuit can make legs appear longer.

• Create interest up top: Stripes or light colors by the bosom take the focus away from heavy or very thin legs.

• Shaving: With an electric razor, use powder if skin is damp. With a blade, splash legs lavishly with hot water for two minutes. Add a thin film of moisturizer to the wet skin to ease the glide of the blade, then apply shaving foam. Wait one minute and begin. This takes longer than soap. So what? The shave will be gentle and the skin will look better. Flaky legs with nicks and cuts are not appealing.

## Anti-Grub Knee Rub

Grubby, dry knee skin can be greatly alleviated by this recipe. The lemon juice acts as a mild skin lightener and the almond meal helps cleanse the ground-in dirt. The honey softens the skin. No excuse now for dry knees.

1 tsp. lemon juice
1 tsp. olive oil
1 tsp. honey
1 tsp. almond or cornmeal

Mix ingredients well. Rub into knees, massaging thoroughly. If there's any left over, use it on your feet. Rinse with cold water.

## Bruises

Vitamin C should be increased if you seem to bruise easily. This formula is to help remove discoloration.

1 part cayenne pepper
1 part glycerine

Mix. Apply with cotton balls.

*Caution: Avoid eyes and mucous membranes!*

## Honey Soft-Skin Facial for the Legs

1 tsp. honey
1 tsp. milk or cream
1 egg white

Beat the ingredients together until frothy and apply to a clean skin. Leave this on for 30 minutes, or just until it feels dry and flaky, whichever you have time for. Wash off gently with lukewarm water, and then splash on cold water. You'll feel alive and tingly. I once made this recipe with a dozen egg whites, and gave my whole body a "facial." Afterward I washed off with warm water and plunged into a glacial spring—then danced all night long.

## Clay Facials for the Legs

Apply clay and water mixture to legs. Allow to dry. Rinse with lukewarm water. "Facial" clay is available at most natural-food stores. Clay stimulates circulation and tones the skin.

# MASSAGE

Shakespeare said that "Sleep . . . knits up the ravelled sleeve of care," and I'd have to agree, but in my books, *massage* is a very close runner-up. For when it comes to easing tension, aches, and worry out of the body, massage has the infinite capacity to do the job. And it's certainly cheaper than a trip to the Caribbean for sheer relaxation!

Not only is massage very gratifying, but it also helps to prevent injuries caused by overworking the muscles and straining the tendons. This is doubly important for the legs because they house the body's largest muscles and tendons.

An added bonus (as if you needed any more convincing) is that massage can be an aid to exercise and diet in helping the body to shed cellulite. The increase in circulation which brings more oxygen into the area massaged seems to stimulate toning of that area.

Of course, massage alone will not cause cellulite to miraculously drop off by the yard, but it seems too good to ignore.

Years ago, trying to find a legitimate masseuse (female) or a masseur (male) was a trying experience. Unfortunately, massage still has an X-rating because of massage parlors, which *do* offer massage but *not* the kind we're talking about.

Your local gym or health spa may have a masseuse on staff. If not, they will generally be able to recommend one. If your area does not have a spa, a nearby physical-therapy unit or chiropractor may be able to locate one for you.

Of course, don't rule out self-massage. Trading massages with a friend is also a nice idea. A homemade "certificate" promising a massage for a birthday or other occasion is also a wonderful and unforgettable gift.

Several books on massage are available; one of them is George Downing's *Massage Book* (New York: Random House, 1972).

The rule of thumb is always massage *toward* the heart. Anatomical diagrams of the muscles will also help you understand the attachments of the different muscles and aid you in becoming a more effective masseuse. Have fun!

**Massage Oil** _____

    1 cup sweet almond oil
    4 to 5 drops of an aromatic oil of your choice (even vanilla extract is very nice)

    Directions: Apply with caring hands to deserving muscles. Other oils with a deep penetrating action for relief of sore muscles are eucalyptus, cajuput, and arnica.

*Caution: Keep away from eyes and mucous membranes!*

# SUPERSTAR PLANTS FOR SUPER LEGS

    Folkloric medicine has raised the use of herbs to an art form. Herbal remedies for what ails us have survived for thousands of years, and for good reason—they've helped generations of people through what ails them.

    Drugs and doctors were for life-threatening situations only. Even the old herbal decoctions, however, are surfacing in modern times as miracle drugs. For instance, those faint of heart in olden times were given decoctions of foxglove, a small plant with purple flowers that grows by roadsides. Nowadays, foxglove is known by part of its botanical name—digitalis, the famous heart medicine. Mayapple blossoms yield drugs for brain tumors. Botanists propagate pink periwinkle blossoms for two anticancer drugs—vincristine and vinblastine. Inca women of Mexico gathered dioscorea, a wild yam which supplies substances for birth-control pills.

    Herbs are clearly no longer the domain of little old ladies who crochet in front of a wood stove. The various noncrisis aches and pains of our contemporary lives can still yield to the powers of the very plants beneath our feet.

    And the great thing is that you can use herbs inside or outside of you and achieve results. Herbal baths, teas, compresses, and massage oils are all ways to absorb the special properties of each plant. Experiment, and find the superstar plant that's your favorite.

## Super Herbals _____

HERBAL BATHS

You deserve to luxuriate in a bathtub and inhale the steamy fragrance of aromatic herbs—just the thing for your legs, too, after a hard day of exercise. You need a muslin bag or a large square of soft mesh material for the herbs. Mix all the herbs together loosely in the bag, tie the top securely, and then place in the tub. Pour on the hottest water that comes out of the tap—enough to cover the bag—and let soak for ten minutes. Then fill the tub the usual way and climb in. Enjoy yourself! Think beautiful thoughts.

## Relaxing Nerves and Sore Muscles _____

1 handful dried lavender flowers
1 handful rosemary leaves
1 handful dried chamomile flowers
1 handful mint leaves

Any single one of the above or any combination could be tried. For single-herb baths use four times the amount.

## Varicose Veins _____

1 handful dried chamomile flowers
1 handful dried calendula (marigold) flowers
1 handful dried violet leaves and flowers

For single-herb baths use triple amounts. Any combination of the above could also be used.

## General Purpose Mineral Bath

1 cup table salt

Add to bathtub, mixing well. This is how you can use up any salt you may have left in your cupboard—and in a way that's *good* for you.

## Athlete's Foot

Sprinkle some garlic powder in your socks and on your feet. Your shoes will smell like a pizza; but it sure beats having athlete's foot!

Apple cider vinegar is another home remedy. Apply generously to affected areas several times a day, using cotton balls. Allow to dry before wearing clean socks.

## Flaky Legs

Soap dries your skin, and there is no need to lather yourself up as they do in the commercials. Deodorant soap is not only unnecessary on your legs but sometimes contains ingredients that can cause reactions to the sun, like tiny water blisters or blotchiness in sensitive people. Flakiness on the legs can sometimes be eliminated by avoiding deodorant soaps. After all, why would you need to deodorize your legs?

Aloe Vera juice applied to the skin is a simple remedy for dry skin. It's also very soothing and therapeutic on a sunburn or after shaving (as a moisturizer). Works great on your face, too.

## Compress for Varicose Veins

4 large handfuls of dried sage

This is an old remedy used by the American Indians of the desert regions to treat varicosities. Boil for 15 minutes. Then wrap the sage in a cloth, and use as a compress on the varicosity.

## Bruises

Vitamin C should be increased if you seem to bruise easily. This formula is to help remove discoloration.

1 part cayenne pepper
1 part glycerine

Mix. Apply with cotton balls.

*Caution: Avoid eyes and mucous membranes!*

# FOLKLORE'S FAMOUS HERBAL TEAS FOR YOUR LEGS

Use 1 generous teaspoon of your favorite tea to 2 cups of water. Bring the water to a rapid boil in a glass or enamel pot, remove from heat, and add the herbs. Let stand for 5 minutes. Strain it and serve either hot or cold. Honey may be used to flavor and the tea may be refrigerated for use throughout the day.

*Arthritic Pains.*   Chaparral, alfalfa, valerian root.

*Endurance of Muscles.*   Capsicum, ginseng, bee pollen.

*Muscle Cramps.*   Chaparral, comfrey dandelion, alfalfa.

*Pain.*   Hops, valerian root, catnip.

*Scar Tissue on Skin.*   Marigold, marshmallow root, slippery elm.

*Thryoid.*   Dulse. Is used to stimulate the thyroid and thereby enhance metabolism.

*Varicose Veins.*   Oatstraw, comfrey.

# SUPER
# LEG EXERCISES

# REWARDS FOR GOOD BEHAVIOR

At the end of each week, promise yourself a small nonfood treat or some "creature comforts."

## WEEK ONE

Take the phone off the hook, light some sweet-scented candles in your bathroom, fill up the tub with bubble bath, and slink yourself in for 30 uninterrupted minutes of enjoyment. If you have kids, pack them off to the neighbors for an hour—offer to reciprocate the favor, of course. Then revel in the silence while you have it. Threaten your dog with a bath if he even *looks* as though he'll bother you for the next half hour.

## WEEK TWO

Buy yourself a single pink carnation on Monday and another one on Friday. Put it on your desk at the office or someplace in your home that is *your spot.*

## WEEK THREE

Congratulations! You're halfway now. Buy yourself a new red toothbrush—or that new album you've wanted, if your budget allows.

## WEEK FOUR

Buy one of those "stained-glass" stick-on decals for your favorite window. When the sun shines in and you see the rainbow colors on your wall, you'll think of your new promise to yourself, and smile.

## WEEK FIVE

Write HI, SEXY on your bathroom mirror in lipstick. (Yes! I'm serious.) It may sound silly, but even if you are the type who is capable of only Neanderthal grunts before 12 noon, it's still nice to have a happy greeting first thing in the morning. If your kids/husband/roommate say anything snide—*ignore* them.

## WEEK SIX

Buy a beautiful pair of textured stockings in an absolutely smashing color. Wear them and feel *good.* You worked hard to *look* good, so enjoy it!

# MORE REWARDS FOR GOOD BEHAVIOR

- Your baggy "fat" wardrobe that you donate to charity is tax deductible. Get a receipt from the agency. With the money you save on taxes, get yourself a new "thin" wardrobe. By the way, be sure to get rid of your "fat" clothes right away, so they aren't around to be comfortable in, in the unlikely event you start to backslide.

- Work on your tan—it not only makes your legs look thinner, but you *deserve* an hour on the beach or balcony relaxing if you've been working out hard. If you are already blessed with dark skin, take the sun anyway—it's free vitamins and it will deepen your skin color to a more even and richer tone.

- Give your legs a "facial." Recipes on page 23.

- Get a massage—even if it's just your feet. If you don't have anyone around to trade foot massages with, do it yourself. Use some scented oil. Finish with a one-minute wiggle under the bathtub faucet full blast on the *cold.* This is guaranteed to wake you up and keep you going for hours.

# RULES OF THE GAME

Any person can get into shape and start leading a dynamic new life by following a few commonsense rules. Here are the rules:

- *Just stick with it*—being fat can be boring, too.

- *When you're hungry, eat. When you're not hungry, don't eat.*

- *Pick a form of exercise that you like.*

- *Stop reading the newspaper, watching or listening to the news for the next six weeks*—you don't need to know anything that isn't positive.

- After that, when you see the news, say to yourself, "I may not be able to change or control the world, but I can change myself."

- Drink lots of water every day (six to eight glasses).

- Have a special and convenient place for your exercise clothes and gear; if you have to lug it up from the basement each time—you won't.

- Be your own boss. Be ruthless in setting and sticking to *your* time every day for becoming fit.

- Do it with a friend. It's more fun and you're more likely to keep that daily appointment if you know someone else is counting on you.

- Hang up your License to Succeed on the refrigerator—and *succeed.*

# SEDUCE YOURSELF

Regardless of what your legs look like now, remember—you are now in control of their shape. You are doing something *today* to make them look and feel better. Tomorrow you will be able to do more, and so on, and so on. Day by day, as you continue to *do* something, your legs will continue to look and feel better and better, until you will have *super* legs.

Remember, *you* hold all the cards for your own success. *You* decide whether you succeed or fail. This is your project. And don't think you have to wait until the required transformation is complete. Take pleasure in the fact that you are improving yourself right now.

# MEASUREMENT CHART

**Before starting, write down your measurements.**

**DATE:**                                                          _____

**HIPS:**                                                          _____

**UPPER THIGH** (at groin):                                        _____

**THIGH** (halfway between knee and hip):                          _____

**KNEE** (1 inch above kneecap):                                   _____

**CALF:**                                                          _____

**ANKLE:**                                                         _____

# EXERCISES

### Wall Sit

**Purpose:** Uses quadriceps.
**Starting Position:** Feet shoulder width apart, toes pointed straight ahead, feet roughly 18 to 24 inches from the wall (depending on your height).
**Movement:** Lower yourself into a sitting position—back, knees, and feet forming perpendicular (90°) angles, as though you were sitting on an invisible chair. Stay there as long as possible, timing the effort. Try to increase time with each session.
**Goal:** Beginners, 1 minute; Advanced, 5 minutes.

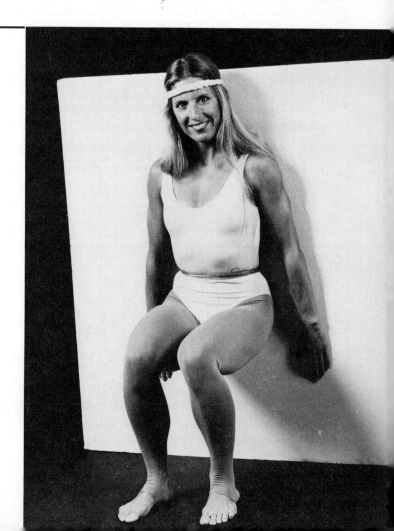

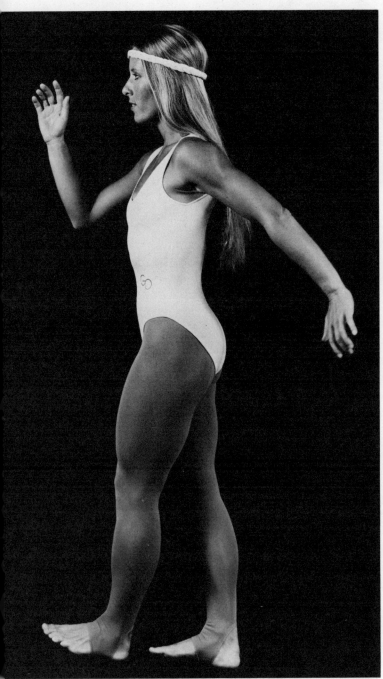

## Toes-Up Walking

**Purpose:** Uses the anterior tibialis (shin).

**Starting Position:** Stand on heels, toes up as far as possible, with straight posture.

**Movement:** Take small steps. Try to increase number of steps each session.

**Goal:** Beginners, 50 steps; Advanced, 200 steps.

## Ankle Circles

**Purpose:** Uses shin and ankle muscles.

**Starting Position:** Seated with legs wide apart on the floor, flex the leg so that the heels of your feet raise up off the floor.

**Movement:** Make largest circles possible with your feet in both directions.

**Goal:** Beginners, 1 set of 30 circles in each direction; Advanced, 3 sets of 50 circles in each direction.

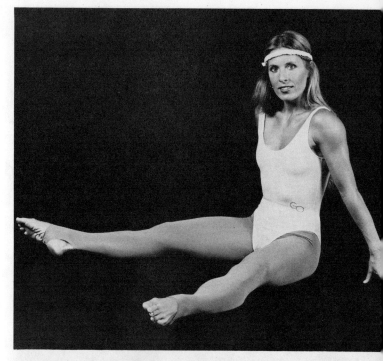

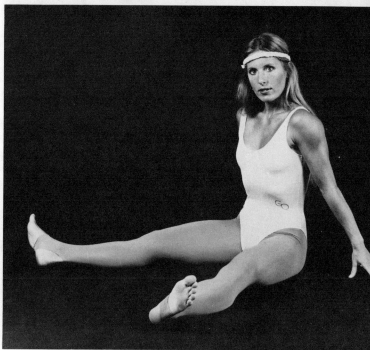

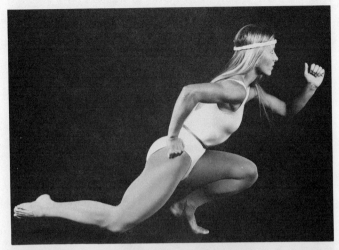

## Walking Lunges

**Purpose:** Uses groin and quadriceps.
**Starting Position:** Squatting, with one leg far in front of the other.
**Movement:** Transfer weight to front leg, then lift back leg off ground. Straighten front leg, while leaning forward. When erect, place back leg in front, lower your body to the start position and repeat.
**Goal:** Beginners, 10 giant steps; Advanced, 3 sets of 20 giant steps.

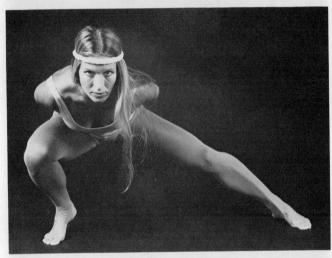

## Stationary Speed Skating

**Purpose:** Uses quadriceps, groin, and buttocks.
**Starting Position:** Stand bent at waist as shown, with legs far apart and hands behind back.
**Movement:** Move body from side to side as shown, being sure to keep the body at the low height of the start position.
**Goal:** Beginners, 10; Advanced, 3 sets of 20. (One left and one right motion equals one.)

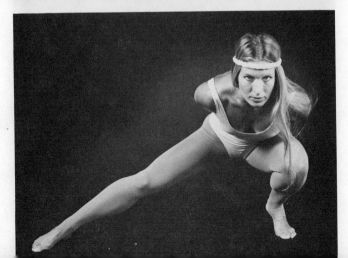

## Scissors with Ankle Weight

**Purpose:** Uses groin and lower hip.
**Starting Position:** Lie on floor face up as shown, with legs together and raised up.
**Movement:** Open legs as wide as possible. Return to starting position and repeat.
**Goal:** Beginners, 20 reps; Advanced, 100 reps.

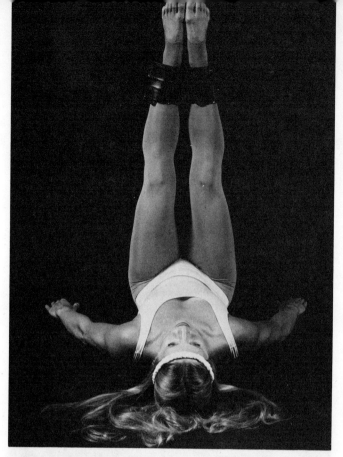

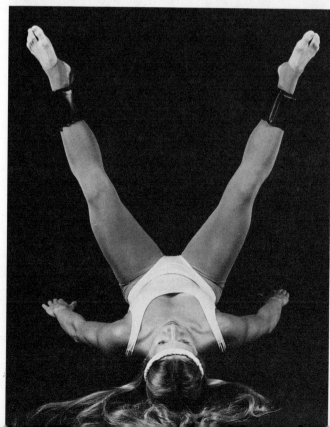

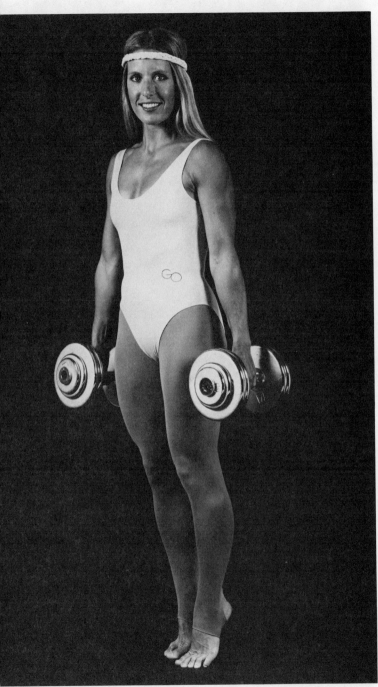

## Calf Raises

**Purpose:** Uses calves and shins. Toes pointed in uses outer calves; toes pointed out uses inner calves.

**Starting Position:** Feet slightly apart, toes pointed straight ahead. Grasp a dumbbell in each hand. The weight of the dumbbell can be quite heavy, as you will not be using your arms to lift it.

**Movement:** Raise the body weight up on your toes. Lower slowly and repeat.

**Goal:** Beginners, 10 reps; Advanced, 3 sets of 20 reps.

## Kickbacks

**Purpose:** Uses buttocks and
hamstring.
**Starting Position:** On all fours,
hands shoulder width apart, back
straight.
**Movement:** Bring knees to chest.
Then kick leg straight back,
sweeping foot high into the air.
Return to starting position and
repeat. Alternate legs and repeat.
**Goal:** Beginners, 25; Advanced, 50.

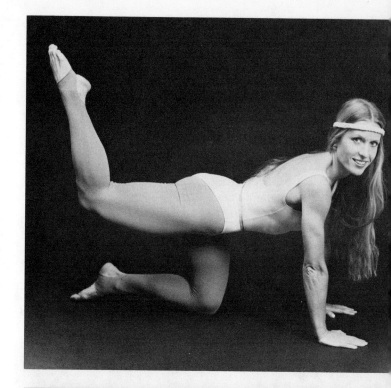

## Jackknife

**Purpose:** Uses lower abdomen and
upper thigh.
**Starting Position:** Sit on floor, legs
together and in front of you. Hands
beside you on floor for support.
**Movement:** Keep legs together,
bring feet off floor. Bring legs into a
V position. Bend legs at the knee
and touch toes to ground. Repeat.
**Goal:** Beginners, 25; Advanced, 50.

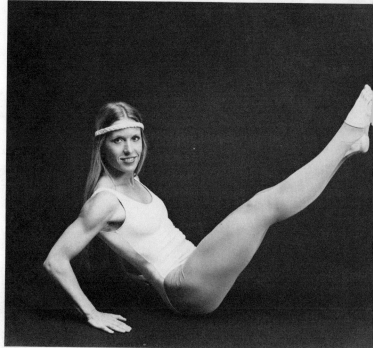

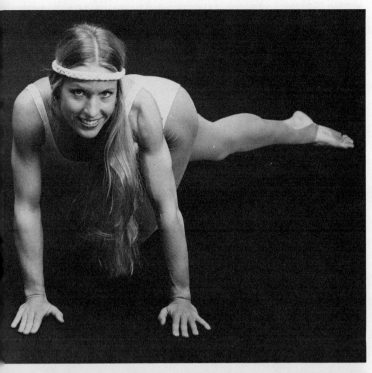

## Hamstring Arch

**Purpose:** Uses hamstring where it inserts into the buttocks.
**Starting Position:** On all fours, hands shoulder width apart. Extend one leg all the way to one side.
**Movement:** Keep your toes pointed, make as high an arc as possible with your toes, bring foot over to the opposite side. Return your leg to the starting position in the same high arc. Repeat.
**Goal:** Beginners, 25; Advanced, 50. (Each time your foot returns to the start position is one time.)

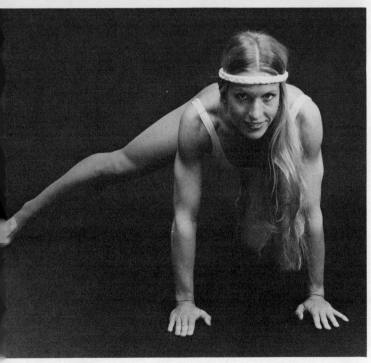

## Sitting Front-Leg Raise

**Purpose:** Uses the front of the thighs.
**Starting Position:** Sitting, legs together and out in front. Back straight and hands to the side for support.
**Movement:** Keeping your leg straight, lift it off the floor as high as possible. Return to starting position and repeat. Alternate legs.
**Goal:** Beginners, 10; Advanced, 25.

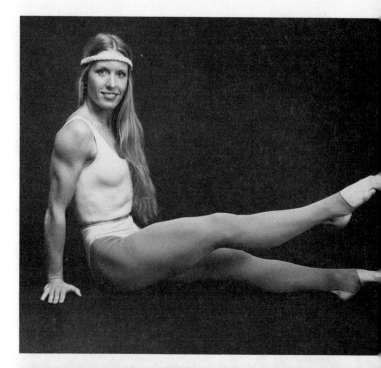

## Backward Leg Raise

**Purpose:** Uses the hamstring and buttocks.
**Starting Position:** Lie on the floor, legs together, face down.
**Movement:** Point your toe and raise your leg up as high as possible, trying to keep the leg straight. Return to starting position and repeat.
**Goal:** Beginners, 25; Advanced, 50.

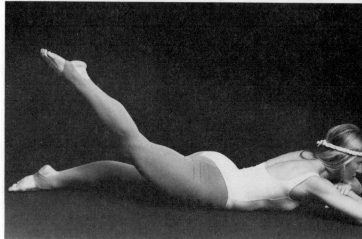

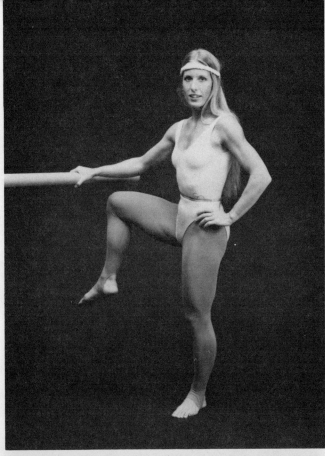

## Groin Brush

**Purpose:** Uses the fascia latae (top of the thigh) and groin.
**Starting Position:** Stand, feet together, hand supported by chair or bar for balance.
**Movement:** Raise your knee toward your chest as high as possible. Then allow the knee to come down, the foot loose, "brushing" the floor with your toes. Raise the knee to the side and repeat the movement. Return to starting position and repeat.
**Goal:** Beginners, 10; Advanced, 25.

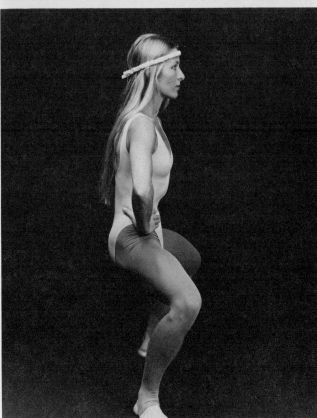

## The Horse

**Purpose:** Uses the thighs and your willpower.
**Starting Position:** Feet apart, back straight, knees bent as shown.
**Movement:** None. Just stay there as long as you can. Time the effort, trying to increase time with each session.
**Goal:** Beginners, 1 minute to start; Advanced, 5 minutes.

## High Knee Sprint

Keep back straight, pump your
arms, and, of course, raise your
knees as high as possible. Take
small steps.
**Goal:** Beginners, 10 steps;
Advanced, 25 steps.

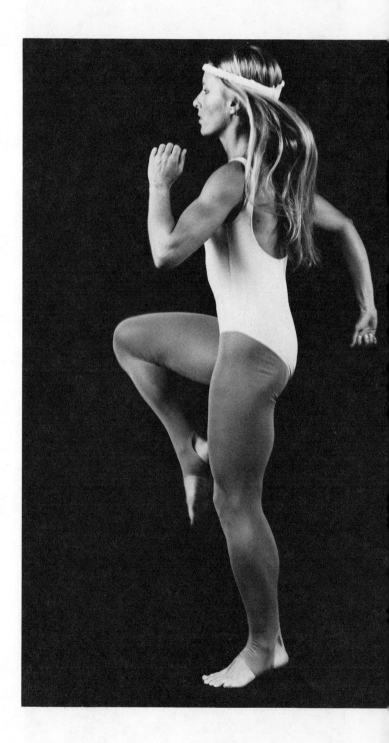

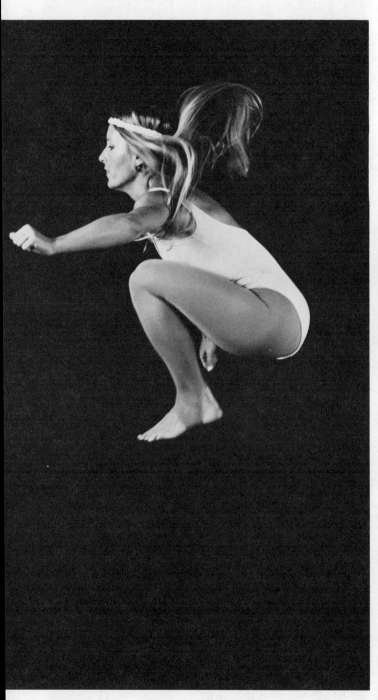

## Kangaroo Jumps

Keep your knees together and try for as much height as possible.
**Goal:** Beginners, 10 steps; Advanced, 25 steps.

*A manicured lawn is a good site for a workout. Kangaroo jumps on the infield at Drake Stadium.*

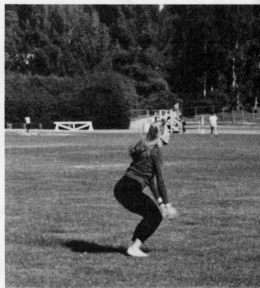

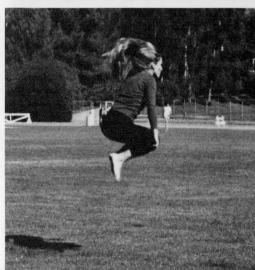

## Hopping

Use a driving, overemphasized arm action. Hop on one leg for the desired number of times, then alternate legs.
**Goal:** Beginners, 10 steps; Advanced, 25 steps.

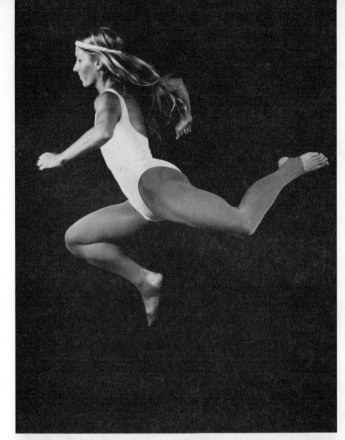

## Bounding

Think of running in slow motion, trying to go up as high as you can on each step.
**Goal:** Beginners, 10 steps; Advanced, 25 steps.

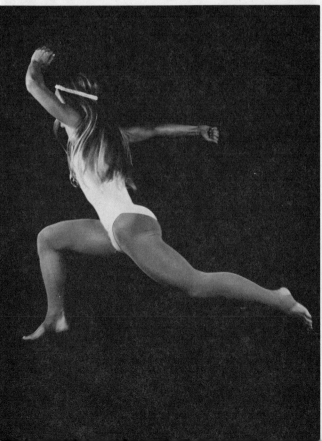

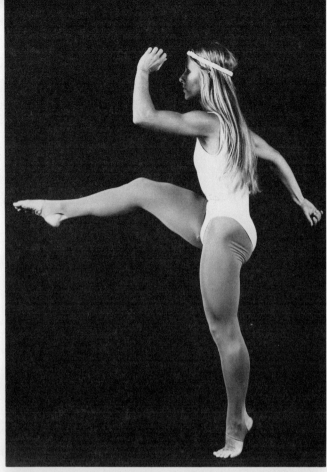

## Skipping March

Knee to chest, moving slowly, arms and upper body relaxed, it's the same way you skipped as a child, only extend the leg in the air before putting it down.
**Goal:** Beginners, 10 steps; Advanced, 25 steps.

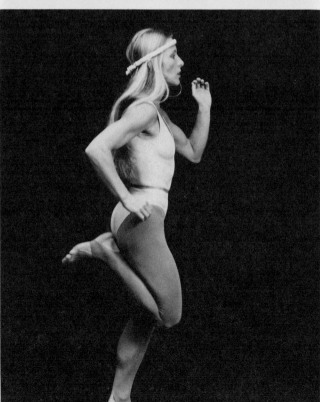

## Kicking Back

**Purpose:** Works the hamstring.
**Movement:** Your heels will actually be lightly kicking your derrière as you perform this exercise. Think of keeping your thighs in a straight line—not allowing the knee to pass the imaginary vertical line from your nose to your toes. Proceed forward in this stylized running form. Each time your starting foot (e.g., your right foot) touches the ground, it's one step.
**Goal:** Beginners, 25 steps; Advanced, 75.

## STRETCHING

My cat, Bambelina, has taught me a lot. Ever watch a cat arch her back and stretch after a nap? Animals know instinctively that a good stretch satisfies like the savory intensity of a good yawn.

Unfortunately, we tend to ignore our instincts to stretch and this can be very dangerous. Stretching helps to prevent injuries. In addition, stretching improves circulation in the muscle, bringing fresh oxygen to a muscle which may have been worked momentarily to exhaustion. Stretching the worked muscle between sets of an exercise, for instance, can allow you to do more work with that muscle.

Stretching is also an inseparable ingredient of speed. Remember that a relaxed muscle that has been stretched is capable of a more forceful contraction and therefore more strength, the result of which is more speed. Think of a slingshot. The further you can stretch back the string, the faster and farther the stone can travel when it's released.

And it's necessary to be able to increase your speed (anaerobic workload) to get the full range of motion from your leg muscles, especially in running. Full range of motion, of course, means that you can maximize your leg development and hasten the arrival of your "super legs."

Need I say more? Start stretching today.

*Lyle Alzado and I preparing for a grueling stadium-step workout*

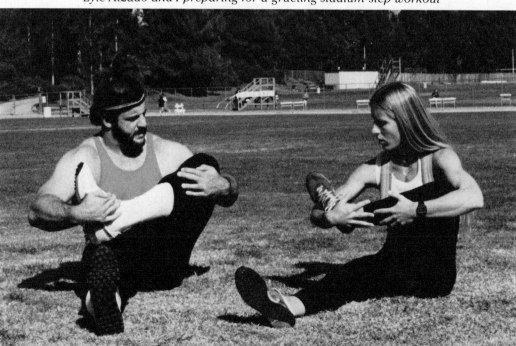

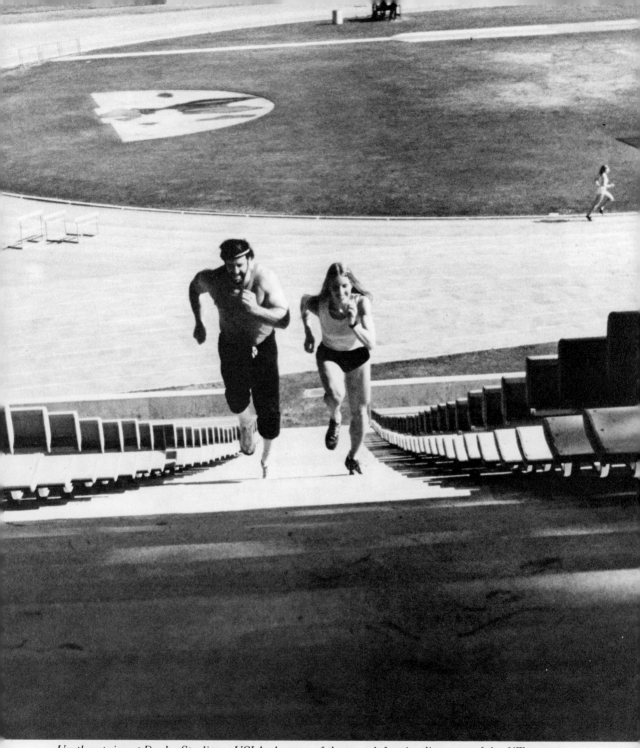

*Up the stairs at Drake Stadium, UCLA. As one of the top defensive linemen of the NFL, Lyle's 265 pounds of solid muscle—and always gives me a run for my money.*

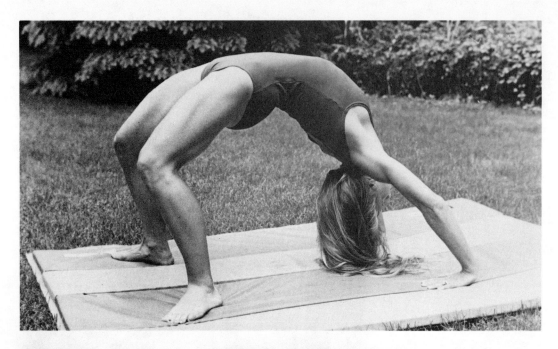

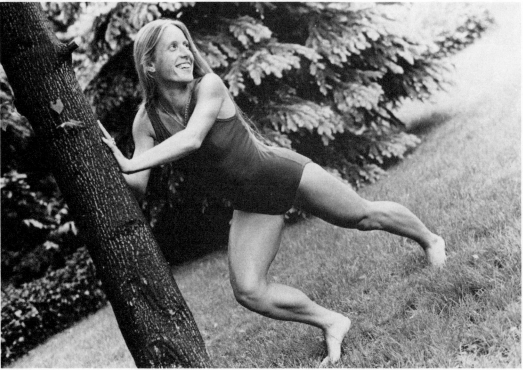

*A good stretch always satisfies.*

## Leg Stretching _____

Hold each stretch for a count of 50.

### Side Karate Stretch

Keep the heels of both feet on the floor. As you become more flexible, move your feet wider apart.

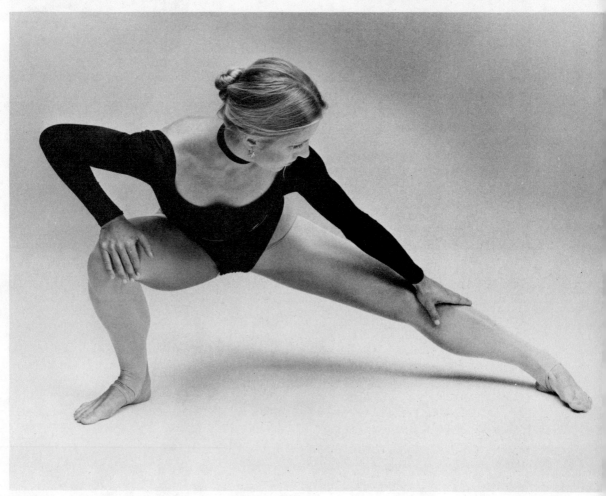

## Reverse Toe Touch

Start in a crouch position, then
straighten your legs.

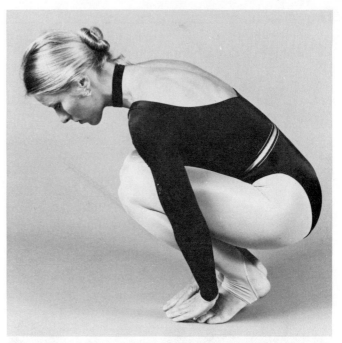

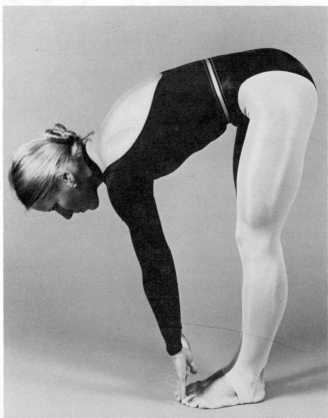

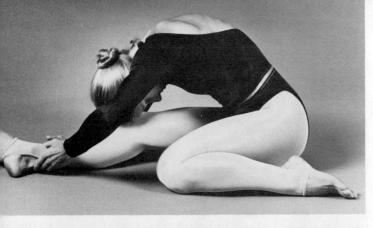

### Parallel Knee Hurdler's Stretch

Go just as far as is comfortable for you—don't force it.

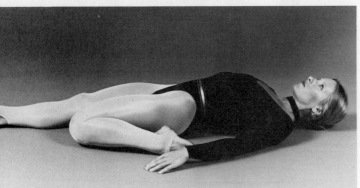

### Thigh Stretch

Simply lie back slowly after you have done the Parallel Hurdler's Stretch.

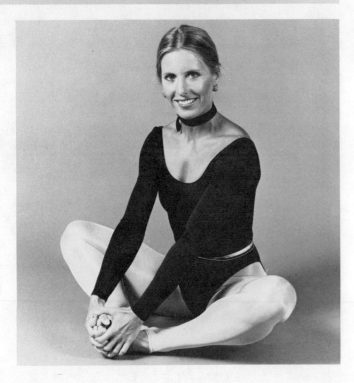

### Frog Sit

Soles together. The object is to bring the heels close to the body.

## Psoas Stretch

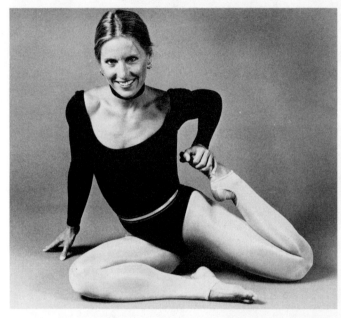

## Calf Stretch

With the back leg straight, put heel
to floor. Then, keeping heel on floor,
bend your knee.

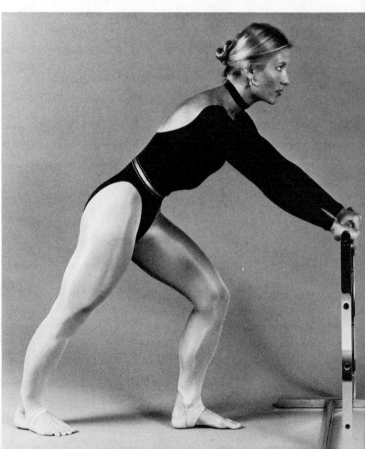

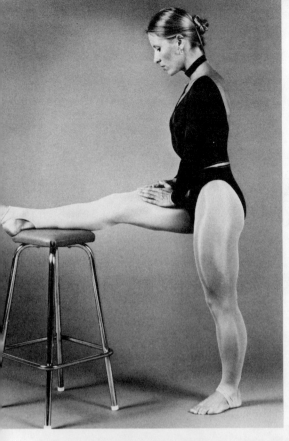

## Dancer's Stretch

You must press your leg down while leaning slightly forward.

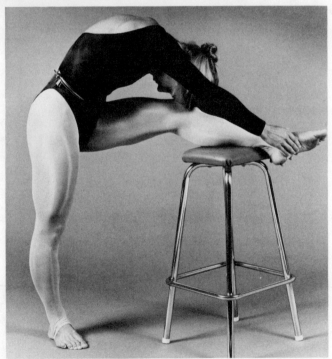

## Hamstring Stretch with a Stool

**Knee to Shin Straight-Leg
Stretch**

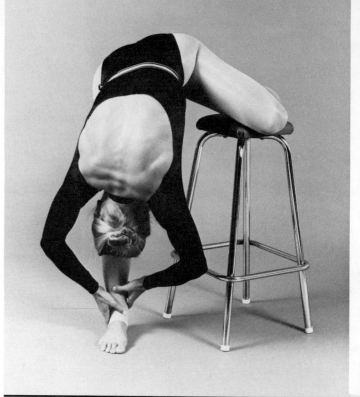

**Salute to the Sun**

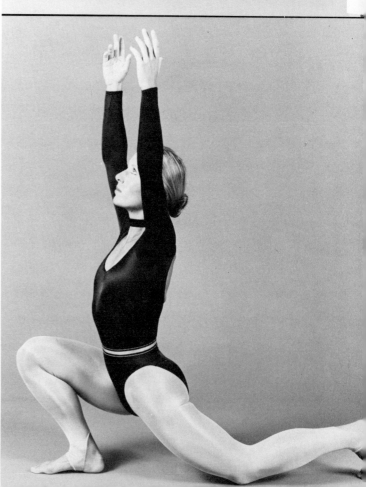

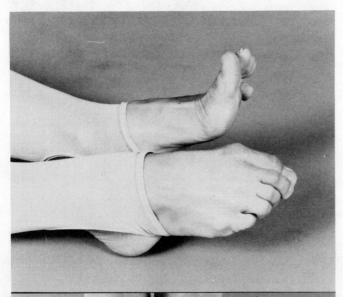

## Toe Crunches

Flex each foot as far as possible in
the up and down position.

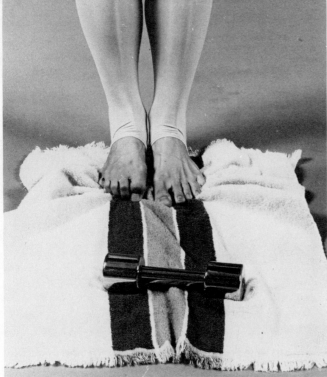

## Towel Toe Work

While seated in a chair, gather
towel with toes.

## Foot Massage

It is not only very gratifying for your feet, but it also helps to prevent injuries.

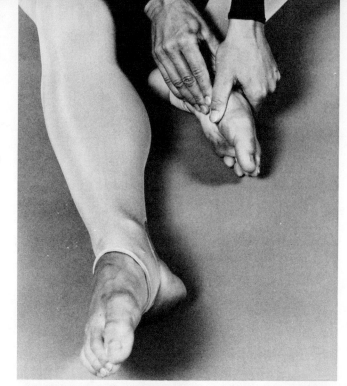

## How to Tie Your Shoelaces

This style of lacing your shoes allows a better fit—enabling you to "custom fit" the shoe. It can be tight or loose over the toebox and arch as desired.

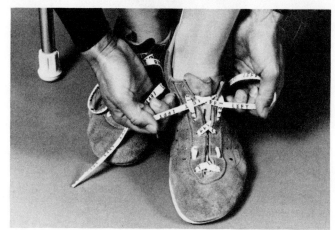

# IMPORTANT:

- Never bounce when stretching.
- Never force to pain.
- Hold each position to a slow count of 30.
- Use stretching as part of your warm-up and cool-down, especially for aerobic activity.

# SIX WEEK EXERCISE PROGRAM

## Chart Notes _____

• Try hard and keep in good form.

• You must keep increasing the number of times you do each exercise. If you want to progress, you must do progressively more each time—even if it's only a fraction more than what you did yesterday—one rep more, or another 30 seconds.

• Start off with a realistic goal, but above the level of mediocre activity. For instance, if you usually walk four blocks, then start off with five blocks.

• Don't rest in between repetitions—return to the starting position and keep the momentum by repeating the movement.

• Move right into the next exercise within 10 seconds; don't waste time on the floor thinking about it.

• The sit-ups are included to help keep your body balanced. Do them bent-knee, do not hook your feet under the sofa or have someone hold them down, as this strains the psoas muscle, which connects to your back.

• Never exercise in sharp pain. This is a test of athletics, not heroics. Of course your muscles may be "workout sore"—this is a good hurt. Sharp pain should never be ignored.

• Feel free to interchange the aerobic workouts—i.e., swimming for walking, and so on.

• Make it your goal to get your heart rate up every day into the exercise range. If you heart doesn't go pit-a-pat, it's not exercise! See pulse rate information on page 76.

• Remember. You must always try harder.

## Week One

**PURPOSE:**
General conditioning.
To get used to doing something every day.
To set standards for yourself.
To establish a base to build on over the next six weeks.
*Note:* Record your measurements and weight on your chart.

**SUNDAY**

| Wall Sit | _____ | *Stretching* | |
| The Horse | _____ | Thigh | _____ |
| Jackknife | _____ | Psoas | _____ |
| Speed Skate | _____ | Salute to Sun | _____ |
| Lunges | _____ | Side Karate | _____ |
| Sit-ups | _____ | | |
| AEROBIC WORKOUT | _____ | | |

**MONDAY**

| Back Leg Raise | _____ | *Stretching* | |
| Calf Raise | _____ | Parallel Hurdler's | _____ |
| Kickbacks | _____ | Reverse Toe Touch | _____ |
| Hamstring Arch | _____ | Dancer's | _____ |
| Sit-ups | _____ | Hamstring Stool | _____ |
| AEROBIC WORKOUT | _____ | | |

**TUESDAY**

| Toes-Up Walking | _____ | *Stretching* | |
| Ankle Circles | _____ | Calf | _____ |
| Kickbacks | _____ | Parallel Hurdler's | _____ |
| Hamstring Arch | _____ | Reverse Toe Touch | _____ |
| Sit-ups | _____ | Salute to Sun | _____ |
| AEROBIC WORKOUT | _____ | Hamstring Stool | _____ |

| **WEDNESDAY** | Toe Crunch | _____ | _Stretching_ | |
| | Towel Toe Work | _____ | Thigh | _____ |
| | Seated Front-Leg Raise | _____ | Frog Sit | _____ |
| | Wall Sit | _____ | Psoas | _____ |
| | Lunges | _____ | Salute to Sun | _____ |
| | The Horse | _____ | Side Karate | _____ |
| | Sit-ups | _____ | | |
| | AEROBIC WORKOUT | _____ | | |

| **THURSDAY** | Groin Brush | _____ | _Stretching_ | |
| | Scissors | _____ | Frog Sit | _____ |
| | Kickbacks | _____ | Side Karate | _____ |
| | Hamstring Arch | _____ | Salute to Sun | _____ |
| | Sit-ups | _____ | Knee to Shin | _____ |
| | AEROBIC WORKOUT | _____ | Reverse Toe Touch | _____ |
| | | | Thigh | _____ |

**FRIDAY**    Rest Day. Warm up for 5 minutes by jogging on the spot, then do all the stretches. Walk briskly for 20 minutes.

| **SATURDAY** | Hamstring Arch | _____ | _Stretching_ | |
| | Kickbacks | _____ | Parallel Hurdler's | _____ |
| | Lunges | _____ | Salute to Sun | _____ |
| | The Horse | _____ | Psoas | _____ |
| | Sit-ups | _____ | Thigh | _____ |
| | AEROBIC WORKOUT | _____ | Knee to Shin | _____ |

You have done the hardest part—you've started! You're on your way now. If you're doing things right, you should have some sore muscles from this honest effort of yours. See your reward for good behavior and enjoy it.

## Week Two

**PURPOSE:**
To improve standards set during Week One.
To build toward the halfway point.
To continue the momentum. By the end of this week, the training will "set" and your body will have begun to change.

| SUNDAY | | | | |
|---|---|---|---|---|
| Wall Sit | _____ | *Stretching* | |
| The Horse | _____ | Thigh | _____ |
| Jackknife | _____ | Psoas | _____ |
| Speed Skate | _____ | Salute to Sun | _____ |
| Sit-ups | _____ | Side Karate | _____ |
| Lunges | _____ | | |
| AEROBIC WORKOUT | _____ | | |

| MONDAY | | | | |
|---|---|---|---|---|
| Back Leg Raise | _____ | *Stretching* | |
| Calf Raise | _____ | Calf | _____ |
| Kickbacks | _____ | Parallel Hurdler's | _____ |
| Hamstring Arch | _____ | Reverse Toe Touch | _____ |
| Sit-ups | _____ | Dancer's | _____ |
| AEROBIC WORKOUT | _____ | Hamstring Stool | _____ |

| TUESDAY | | | | |
|---|---|---|---|---|
| Toes-Up Walking | _____ | *Stretching* | |
| Ankle Circles | _____ | Calf | _____ |
| Kickbacks | _____ | Parallel Hurdler's | _____ |
| Hamstring Arch | _____ | Reverse Toe Touch | _____ |
| Sit-ups | _____ | Salute to Sun | _____ |
| AEROBIC WORKOUT | _____ | Hamstring Stool | _____ |

| **WEDNESDAY** | Toe Crunch | _____ | *Stretching* | |
|---|---|---|---|---|
| | Towel Toe Work | _____ | Thigh | _____ |
| | Seated Front-Leg Raise | _____ | Frog Sit | _____ |
| | Wall Sit | _____ | Psoas | _____ |
| | Lunges | _____ | Salute to Sun | _____ |
| | The Horse | _____ | Side Karate | _____ |
| | AEROBIC WORKOUT | _____ | | |

| **THURSDAY** | Groin Brush | _____ | *Stretching* | |
|---|---|---|---|---|
| | Scissors | _____ | Frog Sit | _____ |
| | Kickbacks | _____ | Side Karate | _____ |
| | Hamstring Arch | _____ | Salute to Sun | _____ |
| | Sit-ups | _____ | Knee to Shin | _____ |
| | AEROBIC WORKOUT | _____ | Reverse Toe Touch | _____ |
| | | | Thigh Stretch | _____ |

**FRIDAY** Rest Day. Warm up for 5 minutes by jogging on the spot, then do all the stretches. Walk for 20 minutes briskly.

| **SATURDAY** | Hamstring Arch | _____ | *Stretching* | |
|---|---|---|---|---|
| | Kickbacks | _____ | Parallel Hurdler's | _____ |
| | Lunges | _____ | Salute to Sun | _____ |
| | The Horse | _____ | Psoas | _____ |
| | Sit-ups | _____ | Thigh | _____ |
| | AEROBIC WORKOUT | _____ | Knee to Shin | _____ |

You are now one-third of the way there! How's your Wall Sit? Are you past 90 seconds yet? See your reward for good behavior.

## Week Three _____

**PURPOSE:**
This is the week to "trick" the muscles into accelerating development.
The intensity must be consciously increased this week to beat those fat cells into submission.
New exercises on Tuesday will vault you onto a higher plateau of shape and fitness.
Get a pair of ankle weights this week and use them in the exercises.

| SUNDAY | Wall Sit | _____ | *Stretching* | |
|---|---|---|---|---|
| | The Horse | _____ | Thigh | _____ |
| | Jackknife | _____ | Psoas | _____ |
| | Speed Skate | _____ | Salute to Sun | _____ |
| | Lunges | _____ | Side Karate | _____ |
| | Sit-ups | _____ | | |
| | AEROBIC WORKOUT | _____ | | |

| MONDAY | Back Leg Raise | _____ | *Stretching* | |
|---|---|---|---|---|
| | Calf Raise | _____ | Calf | _____ |
| | Kickbacks | _____ | Parallel Hurdler's | _____ |
| | Hamstring Arch | _____ | Reverse Toe Touch | _____ |
| | Sit-ups | _____ | Dancer's | _____ |
| | AEROBIC WORKOUT | _____ | Hamstring Stool | _____ |

**TUESDAY** Today's exercises may be new and different to you—something you've never tried before. Remember, if you want to change the way your legs look, you have to be willing to try something different. Do these as best you can. Warm up as per your aerobic workout. Even if you can only do a few of these the first time, that's okay. Next week you'll be able to do much more.

| High Knee Sprint | _____ | *Stretching* | |
|---|---|---|---|
| Kangaroo Jumps | _____ | Calf | _____ |
| Hopping | _____ | Parallel Hurdler's | _____ |
| Skipping March | _____ | Side Karate | _____ |

|  | Kickbacks | _____ | Frog Sit | _____ |
|---|---|---|---|---|
|  | AEROBIC WORKOUT | _____ | Thigh | _____ |
|  |  |  | Psoas | _____ |
|  |  |  | Salute to Sun | _____ |

| **WEDNESDAY** | Toe Crunch | _____ | _Stretching_ | |
|---|---|---|---|---|
|  | Towel Toe Work | _____ | Thigh | _____ |
|  | Seated Front-Leg Raise | _____ | Frog Sit | _____ |
|  | Wall Sit | _____ | Psoas | _____ |
|  | Lunges | _____ | Salute to Sun | _____ |
|  | The Horse | _____ | Side Karate | _____ |
|  | Sit-ups | _____ |  |  |
|  | AEROBIC WORKOUT | _____ |  |  |

| **THURSDAY** | Groin Brush | _____ | _Stretching_ | |
|---|---|---|---|---|
|  | Scissors | _____ | Frog Sit | _____ |
|  | Kickbacks | _____ | Side Karate | _____ |
|  | Hamstring Arch | _____ | Salute to Sun | _____ |
|  | Sit-ups | _____ | Knee to Shin | _____ |
|  | AEROBIC WORKOUT | _____ | Reverse Toe Touch | _____ |
|  |  |  | Thigh | _____ |

**FRIDAY** Rest Day. Warm up for 5 minutes by jogging on the spot, then do all the stretches. Walk briskly for 20 minutes.

| **SATURDAY** | Hamstring Arch | _____ | _Stretching_ | |
|---|---|---|---|---|
|  | Kickbacks | _____ | Parallel Hurdler's | _____ |
|  | Lunges | _____ | Salute to Sun | _____ |
|  | The Horse | _____ | Psoas | _____ |
|  | Sit-ups | _____ | Thigh | _____ |
|  | AEROBIC WORKOUT | _____ | Knee to Shin | _____ |

Yeah, team! You're halfway there. Keep up the good work. Be sure to check your rewards for good behavior.

## Week Four _____

**PURPOSE.**
Now your body knows that you're super serious about shaping up, and will start
reacting faster and better.
Keep trying to extend your limits. This is especially important this week in order to
keep getting results.

| **SUNDAY** | Wall Sit | _____ | *Stretching* | |
| | The Horse | _____ | Thigh | _____ |
| | Jackknife | _____ | Psoas | _____ |
| | Speed Skate | _____ | Salute to Sun | _____ |
| | Lunges | _____ | Side Karate | _____ |
| | Sit-ups | _____ | | |
| | AEROBIC WORKOUT | _____ | | |
| | | | | |
| **MONDAY** | Back Leg Raise | _____ | *Stretching* | |
| | Calf Raise | _____ | Calf | _____ |
| | Kickbacks | _____ | Parallel Hurdler's | _____ |
| | Hamstring Arch | _____ | Reverse Toe Touch | _____ |
| | Sit-ups | _____ | Dancer's | _____ |
| | AEROBIC WORKOUT | _____ | Hamstring Stool | _____ |
| | | | | |
| **TUESDAY** | Toes-Up Walking | _____ | *Stretching* | |
| | Ankle Circles | _____ | Frog Sit | _____ |
| | High Knee Sprint | _____ | Thigh | _____ |
| | Kangaroo Jumps | _____ | Karate | _____ |
| | Hopping | _____ | Calf | _____ |
| | Skipping March | _____ | Reverse Toe Touch | _____ |
| | Kickbacks | _____ | Psoas | _____ |
| | AEROBIC WORKOUT | _____ | Salute to Sun | _____ |

| **WEDNESDAY** | Toe Crunch | _____ | _Stretching_ | |
| | Towel Toe Work | _____ | Calf | _____ |
| | Wall Sit | _____ | Thigh | _____ |
| | Lunges | _____ | Frog Sit | _____ |
| | The Horse | _____ | Psoas | _____ |
| | Sit-ups | _____ | Salute to Sun | _____ |
| | AEROBIC WORKOUT | _____ | | |

| **THURSDAY** | Groin Brush | _____ | _Stretching_ | |
| | Scissors | _____ | Frog Sit | _____ |
| | Kickbacks | _____ | Side Karate | _____ |
| | Hamstring Arch | _____ | Salute to Sun | _____ |
| | Sit-ups | _____ | Knee to Shin | _____ |
| | AEROBIC WORKOUT | _____ | Reverse Toe Touch | _____ |

**FRIDAY**     Rest Day. Warm up for 5 minutes, then do all the stretches. Walk briskly for 20 minutes.

| **SATURDAY** | Hamstring Arch | _____ | _Stretching_ | |
| | Kickbacks | _____ | Parallel Hurdler's | _____ |
| | Lunges | _____ | Salute to Sun | _____ |
| | The Horse | _____ | Psoas | _____ |
| | Sit-ups | _____ | Thigh | _____ |
| | AEROBIC WORKOUT | _____ | Knee to Shin | _____ |

You're two-thirds of the way now! Start dreaming of running on the beach in a racy one-piece maillot. Check out this week's rewards for good behavior.

## Week Five

**PURPOSE:**
To maintain what you've done so far, and prepare for a stupendous windup in Week Six.

To *double* the repetitions you do in each exercise by doing two sets of each, i.e., one set of 25 reps, then wait 30 seconds and do another set of 25 reps.

| SUNDAY | | | *Stretching* | |
|---|---|---|---|---|
| | Wall Sit | _____ | | |
| | The Horse | _____ | Thigh | _____ |
| | Jackknife | _____ | Psoas | _____ |
| | Speed Skate | _____ | Salute to Sun | _____ |
| | Lunges | _____ | Side Karate | _____ |
| | Sit-ups | _____ | | |
| | AEROBIC WORKOUT | _____ | | |

| MONDAY | | | *Stretching* | |
|---|---|---|---|---|
| | Back Leg Raise | _____ | | |
| | Calf Raise | _____ | Calf | _____ |
| | Kickbacks | _____ | Parallel Hurdler's | _____ |
| | Hamstring Arch | _____ | Reverse Toe Touch | _____ |
| | Sit-ups | _____ | Dancer's | _____ |
| | AEROBIC WORKOUT | _____ | Hamstring Stool | _____ |

| TUESDAY | | | *Stretching* | |
|---|---|---|---|---|
| | High Knee Sprint | _____ | | |
| | Kangaroo Jumps | _____ | Calf | _____ |
| | Hopping | _____ | Parallel Hurdler's | _____ |
| | Skipping March | _____ | Reverse Toe Touch | _____ |
| | Kickbacks | _____ | Salute to Sun | _____ |
| | AEROBIC WORKOUT | _____ | Hamstring Stool | _____ |

*Note:* Don't forget to do two sets of everything today.

| WEDNESDAY | Toe Crunch | _____ | *Stretching* | |
|---|---|---|---|---|
| | Towel Toe Work | _____ | Thigh | _____ |
| | Seated Front-Leg Raise | _____ | Frog Sit | _____ |
| | Wall Sit | _____ | Psoas | _____ |
| | Lunges | _____ | Salute to Sun | _____ |
| | The Horse | _____ | Side Karate | _____ |
| | Sit-ups | _____ | | |
| | AEROBIC WORKOUT | _____ | | |

| THURSDAY | Groin Brush | _____ | *Stretching* | |
|---|---|---|---|---|
| | Scissors | _____ | Frog Sit | _____ |
| | Kickbacks | _____ | Side Karate | _____ |
| | Hamstring Arch | _____ | Salute to Sun | _____ |
| | Sit-ups | _____ | Knee to Shin | _____ |
| | AEROBIC WORKOUT | _____ | Reverse Toe Touch | _____ |
| | | | Thigh | _____ |

**FRIDAY**    Rest Day—and you deserve it! Warm up for 5 minutes, then do all the stretches. Walk briskly for 20 minutes.

| SATURDAY | Hamstring Arch | _____ | *Stretching* | |
|---|---|---|---|---|
| | Kickbacks | _____ | Parallel Hurdler's | _____ |
| | Lunges | _____ | Salute to Sun | _____ |
| | The Horse | _____ | Psoas | _____ |
| | Sit-ups | _____ | Thigh | _____ |
| | AEROBIC WORKOUT | _____ | Knee to Shin | _____ |

This was a hard week, but you *did it!* Just one more week to your "graduation." Check your rewards for good behavior.

## Week Six

**PURPOSE:**
To achieve a stupendous wind-up for your program.
Really go for it this week!
Goal for Wall Sit—try for 5 minutes.
Go for 3 sets of the exercises this week.

| **SUNDAY** | Wall Sit | _____ | _Stretching_ | |
| | The Horse | _____ | Thigh | _____ |
| | Jackknife | _____ | Psoas | _____ |
| | Speed Skate | _____ | Salute to Sun | _____ |
| | Sit-ups | _____ | Side Karate | _____ |
| | Lunges | _____ | Calf | _____ |
| | AEROBIC WORKOUT | _____ | | |
| | | | | |
| **MONDAY** | Back Leg Raise | _____ | _Stretching_ | |
| | Calf Raise | _____ | Calf | _____ |
| | Kickbacks | _____ | Parallel Hurdler's | _____ |
| | Hamstring Arch | _____ | Reverse Toe Touch | _____ |
| | Sit-ups | _____ | Dancer's | _____ |
| | AEROBIC WORKOUT | _____ | Hamstring Stool | _____ |
| | | | | |
| **TUESDAY** | Toes-Up Walking | _____ | _Stretching_ | |
| | High Knee Sprint | _____ | Frog Sit | _____ |
| | Kangaroo Jumps | _____ | Thigh | _____ |
| | Skipping March | _____ | Psoas | _____ |
| | Kickbacks | _____ | Salute to Sun | _____ |
| | AEROBIC WORKOUT | _____ | Calf | _____ |
| | | | Parallel Hurdler's | _____ |
| | | | Side Karate | _____ |

_Note:_ Don't forget—three sets of everything this week.

**WEDNESDAY**   Toe Crunch    _____    *Stretching*

| | | |
|---|---|---|
| Towel Toe Work | _____ | Thigh     _____ |
| Seated Front-Leg Raise | _____ | Frog Sit     _____ |
| Wall Sit | _____ | Psoas     _____ |
| Lunges | _____ | Salute to Sun     _____ |
| The Horse | _____ | Side Karate     _____ |
| Sit-ups | _____ | Calf     _____ |
| AEROBIC WORKOUT | _____ | |

**THURSDAY**   Groin Brush    _____    *Stretching*

| | | |
|---|---|---|
| Scissors | _____ | Frog Sit     _____ |
| Kickbacks | _____ | Side Karate     _____ |
| Hamstring Arch | _____ | Salute to Sun     _____ |
| Sit-ups | _____ | Knee to Shin     _____ |
| AEROBIC WORKOUT | _____ | Reverse Toe Touch     _____ |
| | | Thigh     _____ |

**FRIDAY**   Rest Day. Warm up for 5 minutes, then do all the stretching. Walk briskly for 30 minutes.

**SATURDAY**   Hamstring Arch    _____    *Stretching*

| | | |
|---|---|---|
| Kickbacks | _____ | Parallel Hurdler's     _____ |
| Lunges | _____ | Salute to Sun     _____ |
| The Horse | _____ | Psoas     _____ |
| Sit-ups | _____ | Thigh     _____ |
| AEROBIC WORKOUT | _____ | Knee to Shin     _____ |

*Congratulations! You did it!* Record measurements on your chart. See Rewards for Good Behavior, and enjoy yourself. You deserve it!

## Week Seven

You weren't going to stop *now*, were you? Go back to Week Six and begin again.

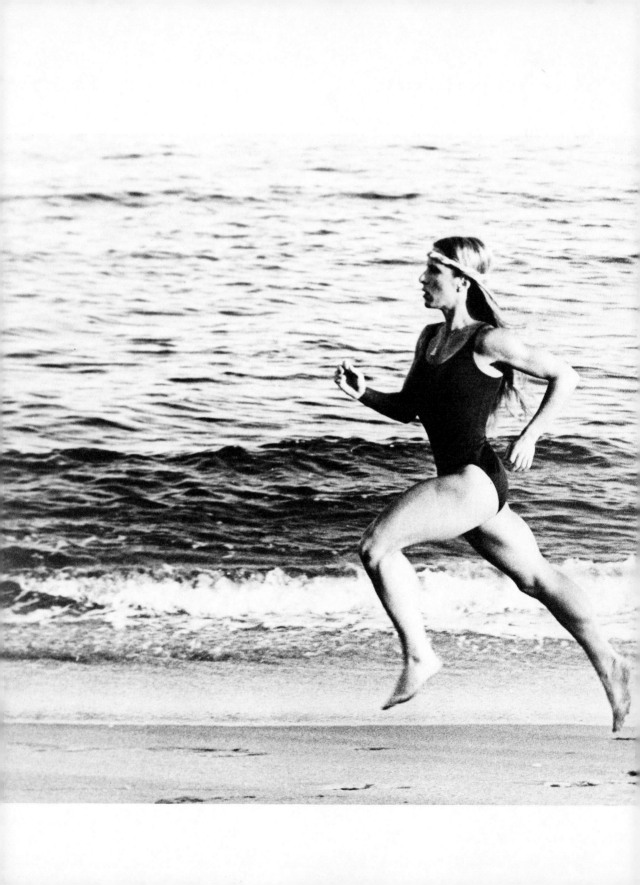

# AEROBIC WORKOUTS FOR SUPER LEGS

# AEROBICS: EXERCISING YOUR HEART

This is how you *burn fat* off your body. The only other way is to starve yourself. You'll be amazed at how much easier it is just to cut out the obvious bad stuff in your diet and combine that action with some aerobic activity every day. Soon you'll discover that you don't even *want* to eat the junk food that invites those little fat cells in your body to bulge you out of shape.

While exercising with ankle weights and calisthenics will give your skeletal muscles the opportunity to get stronger, the effect upon your heart is not enough for necessary cardiovascular fitness. You must also do some kind of activity that enables your heart to beat faster and become stronger. This is called exercising *aerobically,* and it is the premier way to lose weight and shape up.

Pick an activity that you like and then do it. Aerobic exercise does *not* have to be a grit-your-teeth experience. Sign up for an aerobic dance class. After an hour of vigorous moving around to music, you'll be tired, but happy!

And here's another great payoff. When you do something aerobic, of course you burn calories for that time period. However, you also *keep* metabolizing at a higher rate, burning off fat for hours *afterward.* The harder and longer the workout, the more calories and the longer you'll be metabolizing afterward.

That's why it's such a good idea to exercise first thing in the morning or on your lunch hour if you can. This way you'll feel invigorated for the rest of the day. Studies also show that those who exercise before two o'clock in the afternoon are more likely to keep up their fitness program than those who leave it until late in the day.

## How to Take Your Pulse

Immediately upon stopping your workout, take your pulse for 10 seconds in order to calculate the training effect. Then multiply by 6 and you'll have calculated your actual heart rate. Take your pulse directly over your heart on the left side of your chest or under the jawline halfway between the chin and ear.

## How to Exercise Your Heart

The first thing to do is decide which kind of aerobic activity you want to do. Good examples are walking, bicycling, swimming, jogging, cross-country skiing, rowing, and rope jumping.

How hard should you do it? Most experts feel that to achieve a training effect, you must exercise at an intensity that will allow your heart to beat between 60 and 80 percent of your maximum capacity.

To compute your maximum capacity or heart rate, use this formula:

Use the number 220, and subtract your age.
   220 − (your age) = maximum

A mid-range training-rate zone for your heart could be figured out by calculating 70 percent of your maximum.

For example:

If you are 40 years old,
   220 − 40 = 180
   70% of 180 = 126 beats per minute

For convenience, compute how many beats that would mean for 10 seconds; the number is 21.

Now you can take your heart rate for 10 seconds during your workout and know if you're working hard enough.

As your cardiovascular system becomes stronger, your work will become easier and you will be forced to increase the tempo or intensity of your activities to maintain a training effect on your heart. This is similar to the way a 10-pound dumbbell can become too light for your biceps once you become stronger.

## How Long?

The absolute minimum duration is 10 minutes. However, 15 to 20 minutes of honest aerobic activity per day is considered to be very good. Of course, this will not get you into the Olympics, but it will certainly keep you in good shape. Spend a few minutes before your workout doing some easy activity as a warm-up, and a few minutes at the conclusion of the workout as a cool-down.

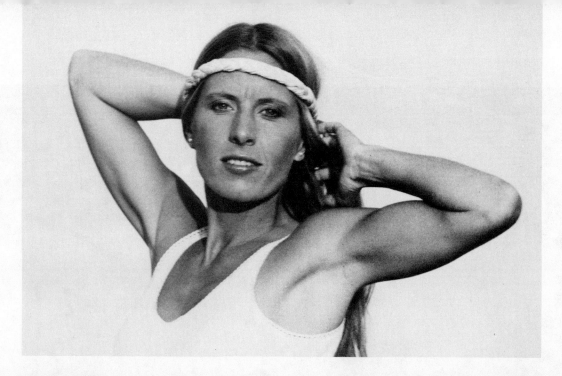

## Making Time

1. Set a regular time for your exercise and let nothing else keep you from this appointment.

2. Find a workout partner if possible. It's more fun, and it's more difficult to miss when someone else is depending on you.

3. Use good equipment. A beautiful leotard or super-comfortable shoes also make you feel good.

## What You Can Expect from Getting into Shape

1. A better shape—a firmer body.
2. A release from stress and negative energy.
3. Better posture.
4. More energy, more vitality.
5. Self-respect.
6. Improved circulation.
7. Better sleep.
8. Better resistance to disease.
9. Good eating habits.
10. A calmer, more positive outlook.
11. Weight loss if overweight.
12. Compliments from your friends and neighbors.

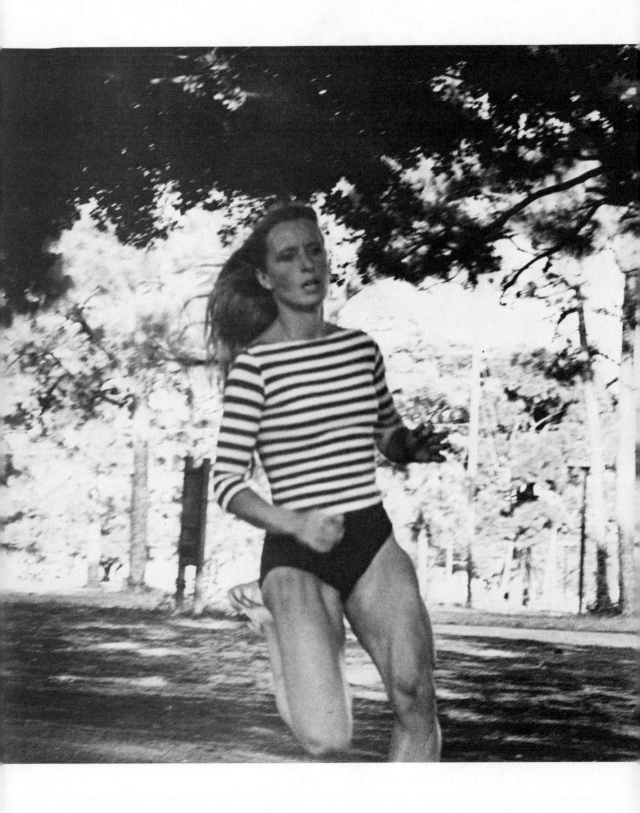

# WALKING

**BENEFITS:**
• Fewer foot and leg problems than from running or jogging.

• You see more scenery than when running.

• You don't need a lot of equipment.

**DISADVANTAGES:**
• You must walk more time to burn the same amount of calories as other aerobic exercising.

**TIPS:**
• Only take Fido if he's trained to stay with you. Kids can be pushed in a stroller and very young babies can be taken along papoose-style in a backpack.

• Strive for good posture and allow your arms to swing.

• Wear a comfortable pair of shoes.

## Program for Walking

*Note:* Window-shopping does *not* count!

## WEEK ONE

• Start with 20 minutes a day (about 1¼ miles).

• Increase by 1 minute every day so that by Saturday you will have walked 26 minutes.

# WEEK TWO

| | |
|---|---|
| **SUNDAY** | Walk 30 minutes. |
| **MONDAY** | Walk 30 minutes. |
| **TUESDAY** | Walk 20 minutes of "resistance walking." * |
| **WEDNESDAY** | Walk 26 minutes. |
| **THURSDAY** | Walk 20 minutes of "resistance walking." |
| **FRIDAY** | Easy Day—see your 6-week chart for today. |
| **SATURDAY** | Walk 26 minutes, trying to walk at a faster pace than usual. |

# WEEK THREE

| | |
|---|---|
| **SUNDAY** | Walk 35 minutes. |
| **MONDAY** | Walk 35 minutes. |
| **TUESDAY** | Walk 15 minutes, then follow 6-week chart. |
| **WEDNESDAY** | Walk 26 minutes. |
| **THURSDAY** | Walk 26 minutes "resistance walking." |
| **FRIDAY** | Easy Day—refer to 6-week chart. |
| **SATURDAY** | Walk 30 minutes, really briskly. |

# WEEK FOUR

| | |
|---|---|
| **SUNDAY** | Walk 40 minutes. |
| **MONDAY** | Walk 40 minutes. |
| **TUESDAY** | Walk 20 minutes, then refer to 6-week chart. |
| **WEDNESDAY** | Walk 30 minutes. |
| **THURSDAY** | Walk 30 minutes "resistance walking." |
| **FRIDAY** | Easy Day—refer to 6-week chart. |
| **SATURDAY** | Walk 30 minutes, trying for speed. |

* Resistance walking: Seek out hills; walk in soft sand or deep snow.

## WEEK FIVE

| | |
|---|---|
| **SUNDAY** | Walk 45 minutes. |
| **MONDAY** | Walk 45 minutes. |
| **TUESDAY** | Walk 25 minutes, then refer to 6-week chart. |
| **WEDNESDAY** | Walk 35 minutes. |
| **THURSDAY** | Walk 35 minutes "resistance walking." |
| **FRIDAY** | Easy Day—refer to 6-week chart. |
| **SATURDAY** | Walk 35 minutes—really move out. |

## WEEK SIX

| | |
|---|---|
| **SUNDAY** | Walk 60 minutes. |
| **MONDAY** | Walk 50 minutes. |
| **TUESDAY** | Walk 30 minutes, then refer to 6-week chart. |
| **WEDNESDAY** | Walk 40 minutes. |
| **THURSDAY** | Walk 40 minutes "resistance walking." |
| **FRIDAY** | Easy Day—refer to 6-week chart. |
| **SATURDAY** | Walk 40 minutes and really go for it! |

# SWIMMING

**BENEFITS:**
• Uses all major muscles.

• Water's buoyancy takes pressure off joints.

• Free massage from the water resistance.

**DISADVANTAGES:**
• Requires a pool, ocean, or lake and the ability to swim.

*Note:* Do the Sunday workout every day, adding the amounts shown on the following days.

## WEEK ONE

| | |
|---|---|
| **SUNDAY** | **A.** Swim slowly one pool length with breaststroke or sidestroke.<br>**B.** Using a kickboard, flutter kick for 5 minutes.<br>**C.** Swim 1 length with front stroke. Return with breaststroke. Repeat for 8 minutes.<br>**D.** Kick for 2 minutes warm-down. |

| | |
|---|---|
| **MONDAY** | Increase Part **A** one lap; Part **D** 1 minute. |
| **TUESDAY** | Increase **A** to 3 lengths and **D** to 4 minutes. |
| **WEDNESDAY** | Same as Tuesday, but increase **B** 1 minute. |
| **THURSDAY** | Same as Tuesday, but increase **B** 2 minutes. |
| **FRIDAY** | No swimming—refer to 6-week chart. |
| **SATURDAY** | **A.** Do 4 lengths.<br>**B.** Do 8 minutes.<br>**C.** Do 9 minutes.<br>**D.** Do 5 minutes. |

## WEEK TWO

| | |
|---|---|
| **SUNDAY** | **A.** Flutter kick 5 minutes.<br>**B.** Swim 2 lengths (out and back) with front stroke. Swim 1 length breaststroke. Repeat for 15 minutes.<br>**C.** Float on your back, kicking only, for 5 minutes. |

| | |
|---|---|
| **MONDAY** | **A.** Increase 1 minute. |
| **TUESDAY** | **A.** Increase to 7 minutes. |
| **WEDNESDAY** | **A.** Do 8 minutes; **C**—do 6 minutes. |
| **THURSDAY** | **A.** Do 8 minutes; **C**—do 7 minutes. |
| **FRIDAY** | No swimming—refer to 6-week chart. |
| **SATURDAY** | Same as Thursday, but try for a more vigorous tempo. |

## WEEK THREE

**SUNDAY**
    **A.** "Dolphin" kick for 5 minutes with kickboard. This is a type of kick where you pretend your feet are tied together at your ankles, and you kick both legs at the same time.
    **B.** Swim with front stroke for 15 minutes.
    **C.** Flutter kick with kickboard for 5 minutes.

**MONDAY**     **A.** Do 6 minutes; **C**—do 6 minutes.
**TUESDAY**     Swim one-half of Sunday's workout. Then see 6-week chart.
**WEDNESDAY**     **A.** Do 7 minutes; **C**—do 7 minutes.
**THURSDAY**     **A.** Do 8 minutes; **C**—do 8 minutes.
**FRIDAY**     No swimming—refer to 6-week chart.
**SATURDAY**     Same as Thursday, but try for a more vigorous tempo.

## WEEK FOUR

**SUNDAY**
    **A.** Swim with backstroke for 5 minutes.
    **B.** Swim with front stroke for 15 minutes, pushing your pace, or "surging" every third length.
    **C.** Dolphin kick for 10 minutes.

**MONDAY**     **A.** Do 6 minutes; **C**—do 11 minutes.
**TUESDAY**     **A.** Do 5 minutes; **B**—15 minutes at steady pace.
    **C.** Flutter kick 3 minutes. Refer to 6-week chart for additional information.
**WEDNESDAY**     **A.** Do 7 minutes; **B**—same as Sunday.
    **C.** Dolphin kick 6 minutes. Flutter kick 5 minutes.
**THURSDAY**     Same as Wednesday, except 1 more minute of dolphin and flutter kick.
**FRIDAY**     No swimming—see 6-week chart.
**SATURDAY**     **A.** Do 7 minutes, with surging every third length.
    **B.** Same as Sunday.
    **C.** Flutter kick 7 minutes; dolphin kick 6 minutes.

## WEEK FIVE

**SUNDAY**      **A.** Flutter kick 5 minutes; frog kick 5 minutes.
                **B.** Swim 2 lengths front stroke; 2 lengths backstroke; 2 lengths fast breaststroke. Repeat for 15 minutes.
                **C.** Flutter kick full speed 5 minutes.

**MONDAY**      **A.** Do 6 minutes flutter; 6 minutes frog.
                **C.** Do 6 minutes.
**TUESDAY**     **A.** Do 3 minutes each.
                **B.** Do 15 minutes steady pace.
                **C.** Do 3 minutes. See 6-week chart.
**WEDNESDAY**   **A.** Do 7 minutes each; **D**—dolphin kick 5 minutes.
**THURSDAY**    **A.** Do 8 minutes each; **D**—dolphin kick 5 minutes.
**FRIDAY**      No swimming—see 6-week chart.
**SATURDAY**    **A.** Do 8 minutes each.
                **B.** Same as Sunday.
                **C.** Flutter kick 8 minutes fast.
                **D.** Dolphin kick 5 minutes fast.

## WEEK SIX

**SUNDAY**      **A.** Flutter kick 6 minutes; frog kick 6 minutes.
                **B.** Do 15 minutes front stroke, surging every other length.
                **C.** Flutter kick 6 minutes; dolphin kick 6 minutes.

**MONDAY**      **A.** Do 7 minutes flutter and frog kick.
                **B.** Do 16 minutes.
                **C.** Do 7 minutes.
**TUESDAY**     **A.** Do 3 minutes each.
                **B.** Do 15 minutes steady pace.
                **C.** Do 3 minutes each. See 6-week chart.
**WEDNESDAY**   **A.** Do 8 minutes.
                **B.** Do 17 minutes.
                **C.** Do 8 minutes each.
**THURSDAY**    Same as Wednesday—try for a more vigorous tempo on the kicking.
**FRIDAY**      No swimming—see 6-week chart.
**SATURDAY**    **A.** Do 8 minutes each.
                **B.** Do 17 minutes.
                **C.** Do 6 minutes each. Then try a "racing time trial" for 2 lengths.

# EXERCISE BICYCLE

**BENEFITS:**
• Can be used indoors in all weather.

• You can listen to your favorite music.

• It is very good for varicose-vein sufferers or people with foot problems.

**DISADVANTAGES:**
• You must be creative in your workouts to keep them from becoming stale.

• You must invest in a bicycle. However, try renting first to see if you like it. Often rental money can be applied toward an eventual purchase.

**TIPS:**
• You must keep checking your heart rate so that you can keep it beating within your training zone.

• Put on some great upbeat music and go crazy!

• Change the location of the bicycle—on a balcony if your apartment has one. Or put it in your bathroom, wear your bikini, turn on all the hot-water faucets, and pretend you are in the tropics.

*Note:* Do the Sunday workout every day, observing the alterations shown on the following days.

## WEEK ONE

**SUNDAY**
    **A.** Do 2 minutes easy pedaling with no resistance.
    **B.** Do 8 minutes pedaling with resistance. Check heart rate several times to ensure it is beating within your training zone.
    **C.** Do 3 minutes backward pedaling.

**MONDAY**
    **A.** Do 3 minutes.
    **B.** Do 9 minutes.
    **C.** Do 4 minutes.

**TUESDAY**
    **A.** Do 4 minutes.
    **B.** Do 10 minutes.
    **C.** Do 5 minutes.

**WEDNESDAY**   **A.** Do 4 minutes with a little resistance (one-half of usual).
                        **B.** Do 10 minutes.
                        **C.** Do 5 minutes.

**THURSDAY**      **A.** Do 5 minutes with one-half resistance.
                        **B.** Do 10 minutes.

**FRIDAY**          Rest—see 6-week chart.

**SATURDAY**      **A.** Do 5 minutes with one-half resistance.
                        **B.** Do 11 minutes.
                        **C.** Do 6 minutes.

## WEEK TWO

**SUNDAY**         **A.** Do 2 minutes easy pedaling warm-up.
                        **B.** Steady resistance pedaling for 5 minutes.
                        **C.** Then once every minute, for 10 minutes total, pedal faster for 20 strokes (a stroke is counted every time the left foot goes down).
                        **D.** Do 5 minutes of chair pedaling. (Place straight-back chair approximately 12 inches behind bicycle. Sit on front edge of chair seat and place feet on pedals with legs extended. Adjust chair according to leg length.)

**MONDAY**        **A.** Do 3 minutes.
                        **B.** Do 6 minutes.
                        **C.** Do 10½ minutes.
                        **D.** Do 5½ minutes.

**TUESDAY**       **A.** Do 4 minutes.
                        **B.** Do 6 minutes.
                        **C.** Do 11 minutes.
                        **D.** Do 6 minutes.

**WEDNESDAY**   Same as Tuesday, but go for 26 strokes in Part C.

**THURSDAY**      **A.** Do 4 minutes.
                        **B.** Do 7 minutes.
                        **C.** Do 12 minutes with 26 strokes.
                        **D.** Do 6 minutes.

**FRIDAY**         Rest—see 6-week chart for today's information.

**SATURDAY**      **A.** Do 4 minutes.
                        **B.** Do 6 minutes.
                        **C.** Do 12 minutes for 30 strokes.
                        **D.** Do 6 minutes.

## WEEK THREE

**SUNDAY**   **A.** Do 2 minutes easy pedaling backward.
**B.** Do 10 minutes steady pedaling with 20 fast strokes every 1 minute.
**C.** Do 8 minutes steady pace pedaling in a chair.
**D.** Do 3 minutes backward pedaling with resistance.
*Note:* If your bicycle does not offer resistance while you are pedaling backward, then substitute chair cycling. Both of these variations benefit the upper portion of the backs of your thighs (hamstring).

**MONDAY**   **A.** Do 3 minutes.
**B.** Do 10 minutes.
**C.** Do 10 minutes.
**D.** Do 4 minutes.

**TUESDAY**   Do one-half of Sunday's workout. Then see 6-week chart.

**WEDNESDAY**   **A.** Do 4 minutes.
**B.** Do 11 minutes.
**C.** Do 9 minutes.
**D.** Do 4 minutes.

**THURSDAY**   **A.** Do 4 minutes.
**B.** Do 11 minutes.
**C.** Do 9 minutes.
**D.** Do 5 minutes.

**FRIDAY**   Rest—refer to 6-week chart for your workout.

**SATURDAY**   Same as Thursday, but try for a more vigorous tempo.

## WEEK FOUR

**SUNDAY**   **A.** Do 2 minutes easy pedaling with chair.
**B.** Do 10 minutes steady pace with resistance, keeping your heart rate in the training zone (with chair).
**C.** Try for a 1-minute "world record," seeing how far on the odometer you can go in this time. Use regular seat.
**D.** Do 2 minutes easy backward pedaling.

| | |
|---|---|
| **MONDAY** | **A.** Do 3 minutes. |
| | **B.** Do 10 minutes. |
| | **C.** Do 1 mile on the odometer for a "world record." |
| | **D.** Do 3 minutes easy backward pedaling. |
| **TUESDAY** | **A.** Do one-half of Sunday's workout. Then refer to the 6-week chart for more information. |
| **WEDNESDAY** | **A.** Do 4 minutes. |
| | **B.** Do 11 minutes. |
| | **C.** Do 70 seconds. |
| | **D.** Do 3 minutes. |
| **THURSDAY** | **A.** Do 5 minutes. |
| | **B.** Do 12 minutes. |
| | **C.** Do 75 seconds. |
| | **D.** Do 4 minutes. |
| **FRIDAY** | Rest—see 6-week chart for your workout. |
| **SATURDAY** | Same as Thursday. Try for a better 75-second record. |

## WEEK FIVE

| | |
|---|---|
| **SUNDAY** | **A.** Do 5 minutes pedaling with chair (medium). |
| | **B.** Do 10 minutes steady pace (regular seat). |
| | **C.** Do 10 minutes pedaling with chair, increasing tempo 20 strokes every 1 minute. |
| | **D.** Do 5 minutes backward pedaling. |
| **MONDAY** | Same as Sunday. |
| **TUESDAY** | Do one-half of Sunday's workout, then refer to 6-week chart. |
| **WEDNESDAY** | **A.** Do 5 minutes. |
| | **B.** Do 11 minutes. |
| | **C.** Do 10 minutes. |
| | **D.** Do 6 minutes. |
| **THURSDAY** | Same as Wednesday. Finish with a 1-minute record attempt. |
| **FRIDAY** | Rest—see 6-week chart for more information. |
| **SATURDAY** | Same as Wednesday, but try for a new 1-mile record. |

## WEEK SIX

**SUNDAY**       **A.** Do 7 minutes medium pace in chair.
                **B.** Do 10 minutes steady pace in chair and resistance (training heart rate).
                **C.** Do 10 minutes regular pedaling; stroking harder, do 20 strokes every minute.
                **D.** Do 2 minutes chair pedaling "racing speed."

**MONDAY**       **A.** Do 8 minutes.
                **B.** Do 11 minutes.
                **C.** Do 10 minutes.
                **D.** Do 90 seconds.

**TUESDAY**      **A.** Do 5 minutes.
                **B.** Do 6 minutes.
                **C.** Do 6 minutes.
                **D.** Do 30 seconds. Then refer to 6-week chart.

**WEDNESDAY**    **A.** Do 8 minutes.
                **B.** Do 12 minutes.
                **C.** Do 12 minutes.
                **D.** Do 3 minutes.

**THURSDAY**     **A.** Do 8 minutes.
                **B.** Do 12 minutes.
                **C.** Do 12 minutes.
                **D.** Do 4 minutes.

**FRIDAY**       Rest—see 6-week chart for more information.

**SATURDAY**     Same as Thursday, but try for a more vigorous pace throughout.

# RUNNING

**BENEFITS:**
• A great way to develop your legs.

• Burns calories (and fat) faster than walking, swimming, or cycling.

**DISADVANTAGES:**
• If you are very overweight, your feet could really take a pounding.

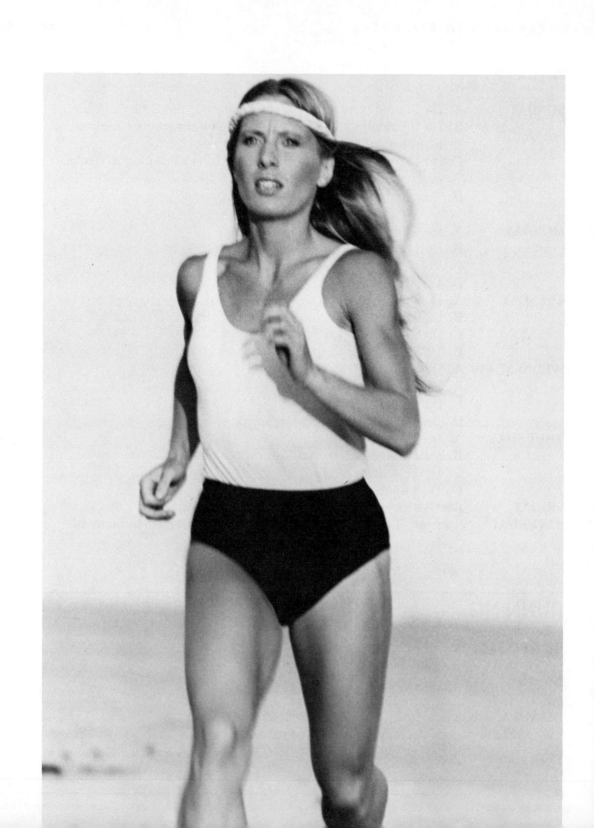

**TIPS:**
• Warm up for a few minutes and stretch before running.

• Buy some good running shoes and keep them only for running.

## WEEK ONE

| | |
|---|---|
| **SUNDAY** | Jog 1 mile, easy pace (approximately 9 to 10 minutes). |
| **MONDAY** | Brisk 30-minute walk. |
| **TUESDAY** | Jog 10 minutes. |
| **WEDNESDAY** | Jog 12 minutes, steady pace. |
| **THURSDAY** | Brisk 30-minute walk. |
| **FRIDAY** | Rest—consult 6-week chart for more information. |
| **SATURDAY** | Jog 12 minutes, steady pace. |

## WEEK TWO

| | |
|---|---|
| **SUNDAY** | Jog 13 minutes, easy pace. |
| **MONDAY** | Brisk 35-minute walk. |
| **TUESDAY** | Jog 12 minutes. |
| **WEDNESDAY** | Jog 13 minutes, steady pace. |
| **THURSDAY** | Jog 13 minutes—try harder last 5 minutes. |
| **FRIDAY** | Rest—consult 6-week chart for more information. |
| **SATURDAY** | Jog 13 minutes. |

## WEEK THREE

| | |
|---|---|
| **SUNDAY** | Run 2 miles, steady pace. |
| **MONDAY** | Jog 13 minutes. |
| **TUESDAY** | Jog 7 minutes, then see 6-week chart. |
| **WEDNESDAY** | Jog 13 minutes. |
| **THURSDAY** | Run 9 minutes, stretch, then speedwork.* |
| **FRIDAY** | Rest—consult 6-week chart for more information. |
| **SATURDAY** | Jog 14 minutes. |

* See page 94.

## WEEK FOUR

| | |
|---|---|
| **SUNDAY** | Run 2¼ miles, steady pace. |
| **MONDAY** | Jog 14 minutes. |
| **TUESDAY** | Jog 8 minutes, then see 6-week chart. |
| **WEDNESDAY** | Run 15 minutes. |
| **THURSDAY** | Run 10 minutes, stretch, then speedwork.* |
| **FRIDAY** | Rest—see 6-week chart for more information. |
| **SATURDAY** | Run 15 minutes, trying harder last 6 minutes. |

## WEEK FIVE

| | |
|---|---|
| **SUNDAY** | Run 2½ miles, steady pace. |
| **MONDAY** | Jog 15 minutes. |
| **TUESDAY** | Jog 9 minutes, then see 6-week chart. |
| **WEDNESDAY** | Run 16 minutes. |
| **THURSDAY** | Jog 11 minutes, stretch, then speedwork.* |
| **FRIDAY** | Rest—see 6-week chart for more information. |
| **SATURDAY** | Run 20 minutes, trying harder last 10 minutes. |

## WEEK SIX

| | |
|---|---|
| **SUNDAY** | Run 3 miles at a steady pace. |
| **MONDAY** | Jog 14 minutes. |
| **TUESDAY** | Jog 10 minutes, then see 6-week chart. |
| **WEDNESDAY** | Jog 18 minutes. |
| **THURSDAY** | Jog 12 minutes, stretch, then speedwork.* |
| **FRIDAY** | Rest—see 6-week chart for more information. |

* See page 94.

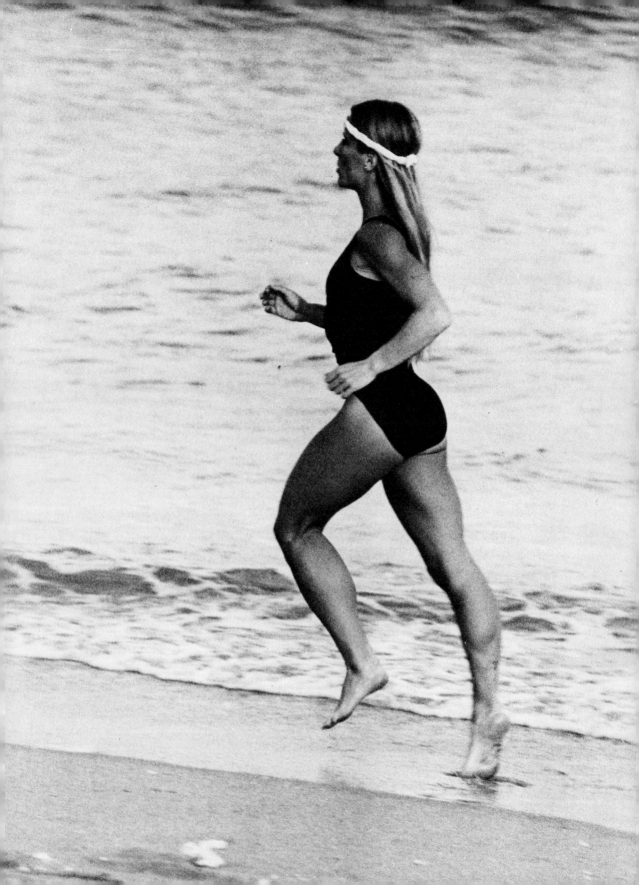

# SPEEDWORK:

## WEEK THREE

Speedwork consists of 10 minutes of jogging, running, and walking segments after your run. Use the distance between telephone poles as your guide. This week, jog the distance between two telephone poles. Then turn around and run the distance hard—then walk *briskly* back and repeat the sequence. Do this 6 to 8 times. The hard-run part should be at about 70 percent of your maximum speed.

## WEEK FOUR

As in Week Three, but use the distance between *three* telephone poles. Do it 8 times at 80 percent of your maximum speed.

## WEEK FIVE

Use the distance between three telephone poles. Do it 10 times at 90 percent of your maximum speed.

## WEEK SIX

Use the distance between four telephone poles. Do it 8 times at 90 percent of your maximum speed.

*Note:* You can substitute a vigorous hour of an aerobic-style dancing class for any of the workouts, except Tuesdays, as that is a specialized leg-development day.

**After WEEK SIX**

**DATE:** _____

**HIPS:** _____

**UPPER THIGH:** _____

**THIGH:** _____

**KNEE:** _____

**CALF:** _____

**ANKLE:** _____

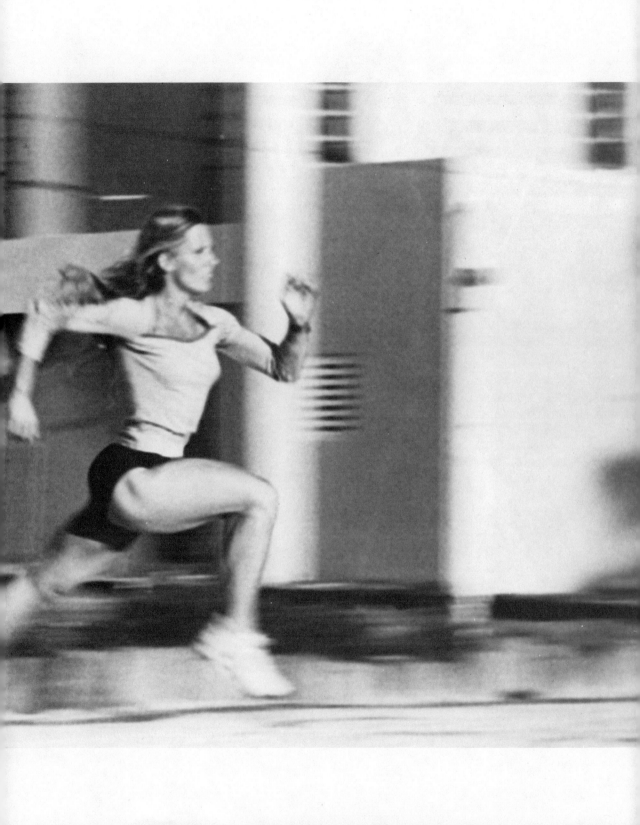

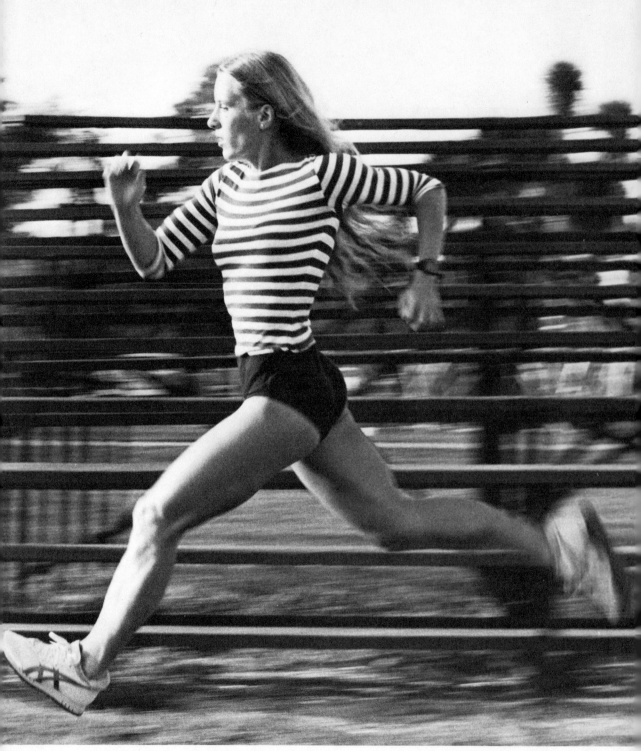

*I always incorporate fast running into my program for complete leg development.*

*Shooting a scene on location. Sunset in the South Pacific*

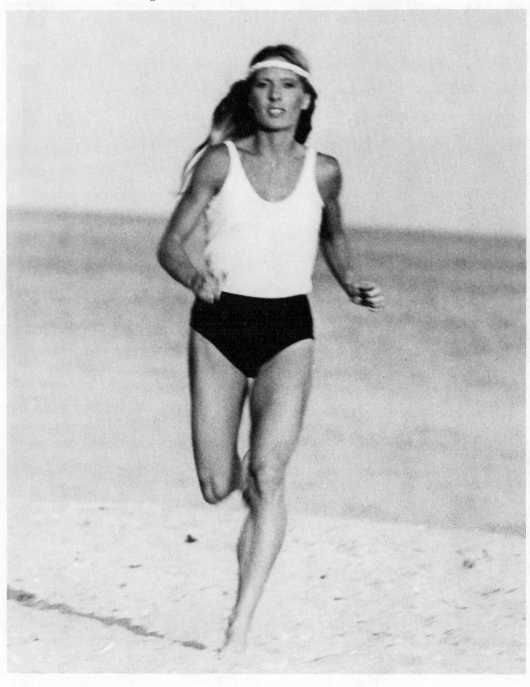

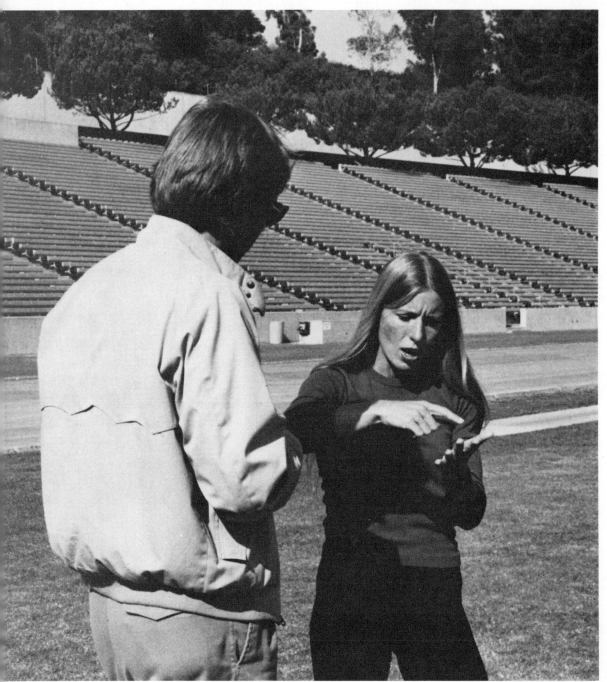

*Questions and answers*

# QUESTIONS AND
# ANSWERS

**Q.** What causes swollen feet and ankles? My neighbor says you just get that when you start getting older. I'm not a senior citizen yet (I'm 58) but I was wondering if there is something you can do about it. My neighbor's remarks really made me feel depressed.

**A.** Swollen feet and ankles are actually a condition called edema. It is fluid retention in the extremities caused in most cases by excess intake of table salt. Even if you don't *add* salt to your food, most packaged or restaurant food today is prepared with salt—from cottage cheese to ketchup to breakfast cereal.

Omit salt from your diet. Flavor foods with tasty herbs and spices instead. Impaired circulation is another contributing factor to swollen feet and ankles. Garters, girdles, tight jeans, and other tight clothing are to be avoided. Are you getting enough exercise? Standing on your head helps reduce swelling of the lower leg. So does sitting with your feet up whenever possible. For your own peace of mind, check with your physician to rule out diabetes or gouty arthritis.

Finally, at 58 you are a young woman, and the idea that you have to *expect* health problems as you live longer is ridiculous. Health is our birthright, something which need not be traded in as the years go by. Take good care of yourself, and have fun for the next 58 years. And please keep in mind that your neighbor's narrow perspective of "age" limits the value of his/her opinion.

**Q.** I think I may have pulled a muscle in my leg when I was rollerskating on the weekend. (I fell.) It wasn't bad enough to see a doctor, but isn't there something you're supposed to do for a sore muscle?

**A.** The physical therapy rule of thumb is ice it for the first 24 hours. Rub an ice cube on the affected area for 10 minutes every hour.

After 24 hours, start with moist heat—a hot water bottle wrapped in a cloth. No more than 10 minutes every hour.

Eating a whole fresh pineapple reduces the swelling by virtue of the proteolytic enzyme with which it is loaded which actually eats away dead tissue! I routinely have the pro football players I coach eat a fresh pineapple right after a game to keep swelling from injuries in check and reduce lactic acid in the muscles. (Lactic acid is the by-product of an overworked muscle that causes the soreness or stiffness you feel the day after.)

**Q.** Does lifting weights and exercising cause a woman to lose her femininity and become muscle-bound?

**A.** The only way a woman can lose her femininity is on the operating table. Of course, if a woman athlete takes drugs (steroids, for instance, which are male

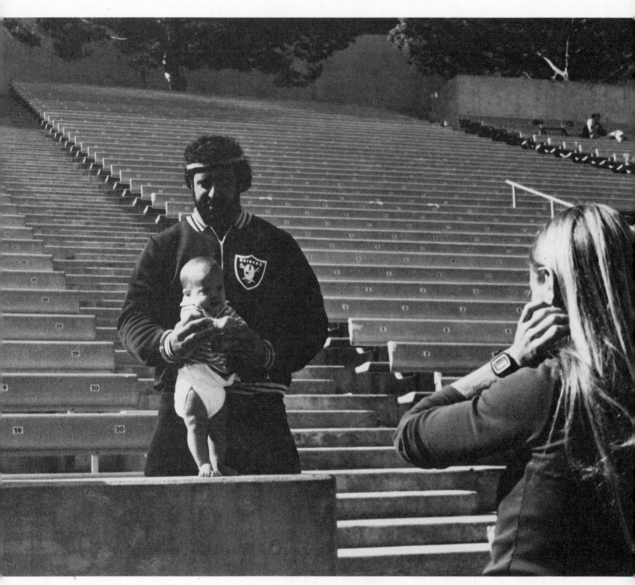

*Lyle Alzado—pro football superstar for the LA Raiders and proud father. I can always count on Lyle for some comic relief after a tough workout. Here, with his son, Justin.*

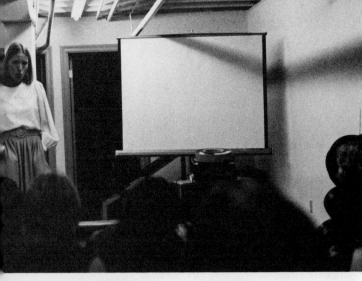

*A lecture, a book signing, and a TV show—as much a part of my day as running, writing, and lifting weights*

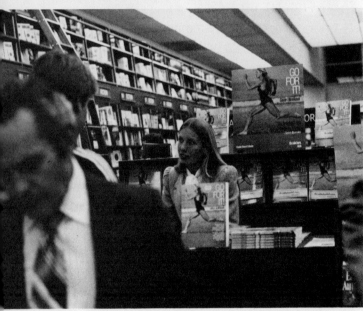

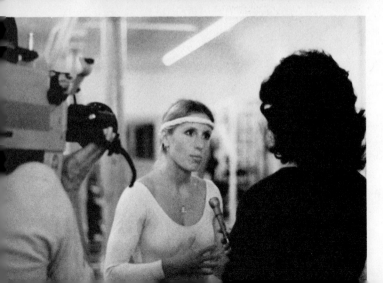

hormones) then that's the same thing as going on the operating table. Frankly, I think more people should ask, "Does cellulite affect a woman's femininity?" It certainly obscures the sinewy, graceful line of a woman's body. Exercising and becoming stronger are the only ways to possess power and grace, and what could be more feminine than that?

**Q.** Speaking of operating tables, what about those operations to surgically remove cellulite? Are they safe? Do they work?

**A.** Elective surgery of any kind always involves risks. The problem here, though, is that you're treating the symptom (the fat) and not the cause: a body whose owner overeats and underexercises. These operations offer only temporary results. Follow the same bad habits and you're back on that operating table again. The only thing that becomes permanently thinner is your wallet. Nature has simple laws which must be followed for good health and a beautiful body. One of the latest fads is a Beverly Hills (where else?) clinic which uses huge hypodermic syringes to actually suck the fat out from under the skin. Of course, the friction caused by this results in tremendous fluid-filled pockets under the skin—actually huge heat-caused blisters. Infection must then be guarded against. Of course, the whole process is certified to be very safe. I mean, nobody has *died* from it—yet. Does it seem like Nature's intention that we should get so out of touch with ourselves that we must pay a fortune to have excess fat sucked out with needles, or sliced off in the hospital? Yeeeccchhh!

**Q.** Does muscle turn to fat after you stop exercising? How do you know what's muscle and what's fat anyway?
**A.** You can't flex fat! Here's the technical breakdown:

|        | *WATER* | *LIPIDS* | *PROTEIN* |
|--------|---------|----------|-----------|
| MUSCLE | 70%     | 8%       | 22%       |
| FAT    | 22%     | 72%      | 6%        |

Should you ever stop exercising, muscle does *not* turn to fat. Without exercise, the muscles may become smaller. If you then keep eating the same amount of food, fat will soon begin to form, but it does not *replace* the muscle; it merely forms *in addition* to the muscle. Our bodies were designed to be moved, to be used, to be exercised. Have you ever seen an obese squirrel, for instance? No. Because animals instinctively follow Nature's laws of movement to survive.

So don't sit around wondering if your muscles will turn to fat if you stop exercising. Just keep exercising.

**Q.** Is there anything you can do to prevent chafing between your legs when you jog? My thighs are still too fat and I get a rash from them rubbing together. It hurts! Help!

**A.** Chafing on the thighs isn't always caused by fat legs. Quite a few pro football players experience the same problem when they run. I tell them to wear cotton sweat pants when they run, or shorts that are long enough to cover the affected area, but tight enough so that the extra fabric doesn't create new problems. Wearing thin leotards under your shorts may work very well. Also, a little oil on the area *before* you go out the door is a good preventive. For the rash you have, aloe vera gel is very soothing. Vitamin E oil also promotes healing. Open a vitamin E capsule with a pin and squeeze the oil on the rash. Incidentally, aloe vera gel and/or vitamin E oil are good for a host of skin complaints—from chapped lips to diaper rash.

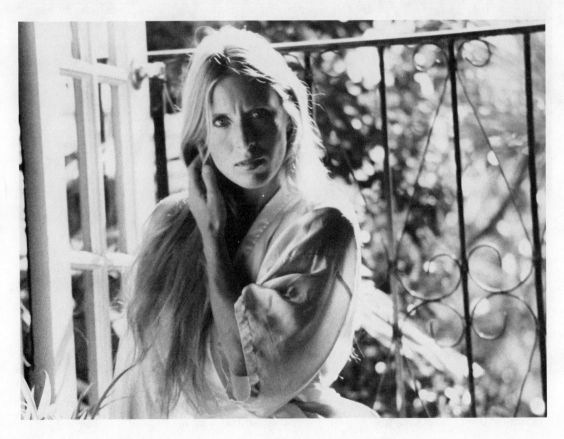

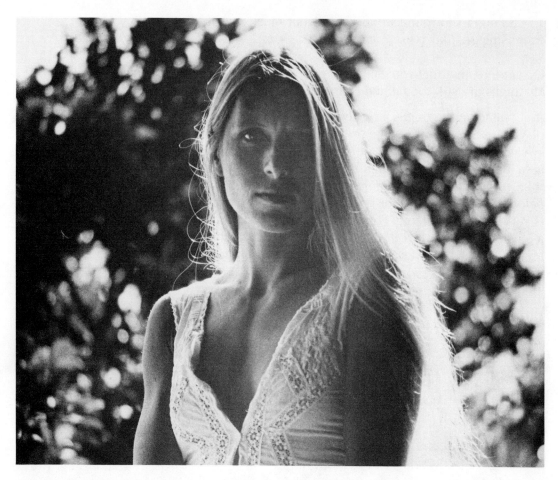

**Q.** Are high heels bad for you? I've been wearing them since I was 16.

**A.** High heels were actually invented when traditions changed, and women's skirts were allowed to be above the ankle. The shorter hemlines revealed "gams," as they were called, which had no shape. After all, how much exercise could a girl get in a floor-length gown? So, to give the female leg a more appealing shape, high heels were invented.

By causing women to walk on their toes, the calf muscles were then always seen in a flexed position, resulting in a more shapely leg.

Unfortunately, this also causes the low back to be thrown out of position, resulting in low back strain and a "swayback" posture. High heels also cause innumerable foot problems. One is the shortening of the Achilles tendon at the heel, including the connecting tendons and muscles all the way up the back of the leg.

If you've been wearing high heels for years, pay particular attention to the stretching exercises on pages 48–58. These are especially important for you. Needless to say, you should switch to lower shoes. Styles are finally abundant in lower heels now as women in business seek comfort *and* fashion from their shoes.

If you do everything in this book, your legs will soon be shapely enough without the high heels.

**Q.** If high heels are bad for you, then those negative heel shoes must be great for you, right?

**A.** They're fine for most people, but approximately 20 percent of the population is unable to wear them because of back and back-related problems.

Walking in a shoe which has the heel *lower* than the toe does give your calf and foot muscles a tremendous workout. However, if you've been in spike heels since high school and decide to go "natural" now, the results could be very traumatic, if not painful. Your muscles and tendons at the back of your legs may have been shortened from the high heels. Therefore, proceed with caution.

**Q.** Is it true what they say about exercise sandals? Can they really help your legs? My legs have always been skinny and I'll try anything.

**A.** Surprise—for once the ad campaigns are not stretching the truth. The exercise sandals make your feet work in a three-part movement when you walk, which not only strengthens them, but also shapes the calf muscles.

You must get used to them slowly. I'd recommend an hour a day for the first week. Then add a half hour every day. Be prepared to walk *slowly*. Your toes are probably unused to doing any work, so you must help them to adjust gradually. After that, you won't even have to think about the feet slipping out of the sandals.

For other foot and lower-leg shaping exercises, see pages 35–47.

**Q.** What brand of sneakers do you recommend? Is there really that much difference between the expensive ones and the look-alikes on sale in the supermarket?

**A.** In a fit of rebellion one day at the elitism of the big shoe companies, I rushed out and bought a pair of bargain basement specials and went running. I ended up taking the shoes off and walking after four miles. Worse, my feet hurt for a week after.

Those cheap shoes may cleverly imitate the stripes and logos of the established shoe companies, but my advice is: Don't fall for it. A pair of super-comfortable shoes for your activity is not only a smart investment in your feet's welfare, but a motivational prop for you as well. After all, you just dropped fifty dollars on those sneakers—you're committed now!

As for brand names, the old adage "if the shoe fits, wear it," could never be more true. Make sure the shoe is designed for your needs, regardless of the brand. For instance, running shoes worn for tennis could result in injury. Running shoes are built only for forward movement and offer no support for the quick lateral movements of tennis.

There are a rainbow of colors to choose from. However, color should *not* be the determining factor. The shoes may go perfectly with your magenta sweatsuit, but if they don't fit your feet or your activity needs, don't get them.

**Q.** I've been doing full squats in the gym for a few weeks now, but I don't seem to see any difference in my legs. Are they good for thinning out your legs?

**A.** Full squats are an old standby gym exercise that involves balancing a heavy barbell on the back of the neck and shoulders, and then bending the knees fully— feet shoulder width apart.

Personally, I've never been a fan of squatting because it is a great strain on the knees, even when done correctly.

I've seen too many athletes end their careers on that exercise. Football players are particularly wed to this exercise, so I advise that if they are compelled to do them, it is best that they *do not* bend the knee fully. A few degrees is enough. These are called half squats.

Also, I've seen greater strength and stamina from other exercises—review pages 34–47. Doing squats also seems to increase the *width* of the derriere because of the muscles used. Needless to say, I don't recommend this exercise.

It's very hard to say something nice about an exercise that strains knees and makes your fanny wider. So I won't.

**Q.** Should you wear shoes for aerobic dancing?

**A.** Remember, you read it here. Get yourself a pair of shoes. All kinds of foot problems are cropping up now from these classes because the feet are unused to the abuse of being jumped on barefoot on hard floors.

There are some specially designed sneakers out now just for aerobics. You need *something* on your feet, not just for support, but also for hygienic reasons (to prevent athlete's foot, plantar warts, etc.). Also, you avoid that "chalky feet" feeling that is certainly unappealing.

Dance slippers, yachting shoes, or canvas sneakers are all possibles—just make sure they give support and are comfortable.

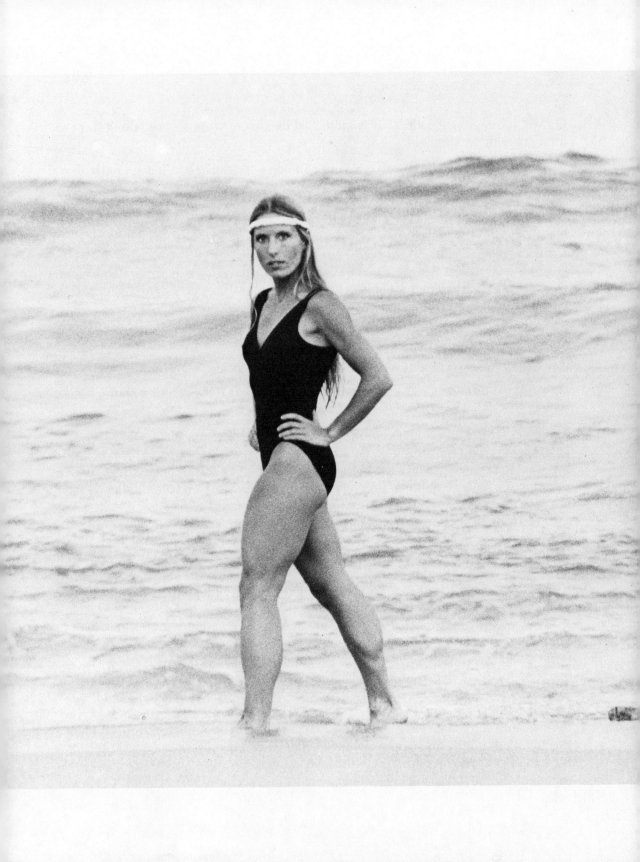

**Q.** Will lifting weights affect my running? I'd like to get stronger but I don't want to interfere with my running.

**A.** Lifting weights definitely affects your running—for the *better.* It's strength plus flexibility that equals speed.

Lifting makes you stronger. You look better, you feel better, you run faster, and you have fewer injuries. Years ago, I was ostracized by some of my competitors because I looked different than they did, due to my lifting. It was against tradition for a runner to lift weights.

Lately, I've read that even some of my former critics have incorporated weight-training into their regimens. I chuckle when I read how they now extol the virtues of weight-training for runners. As I've said for years, it works.

Check out the drills on pages 45–47 and the stretching section, too. This will keep you flexible and add to your speed.


**Q.** I've been running for five years and can't seem to lose the cellulite on my legs. Why?

**A.** You don't say how much you run, over what type of terrain (flat or hilly), or at what speed. If you run slowly on flat ground, your muscle development will be incomplete because you are not getting full range of motion out of your legs. Hence, even though you are running, which is terrific, parts of your leg (the saddlebag sections) are basically getting a free ride.

You're in good company, if it's any consolation. Some world-class marathoners —who have possibly the skinniest bodies in the world—also have cellulite. Why? Because exercise alone is not enough for total fitness. Diet is another very important factor here. Sadly, athletes often feel that because they exercise they can get away with eating anything in the world—including the worst junk food. Review the sections on pages 7–12 on diet and cellulite.

Obviously, your problem would be much worse if you did nothing at all. In addition, realize that running is great, but it's not the *only* thing. Review the exercise section and incorporate them into your regimen.

Finally, trying running *faster.* I have yet to see a sprinter with cellulite. Anaerobic exercising (the stuff that is full out for 10 to 20 seconds at a time) seems to burn off the old cellulite.

Start off with some easy sprinting at 60 percent of your full speed. Sprint like this for a hundred yards (or the distance between two telephone poles). Do this at the end of your running workout, four times a week, ten sprints each time, preferably uphill if possible. Walk back to start quickly between each one. Gradually

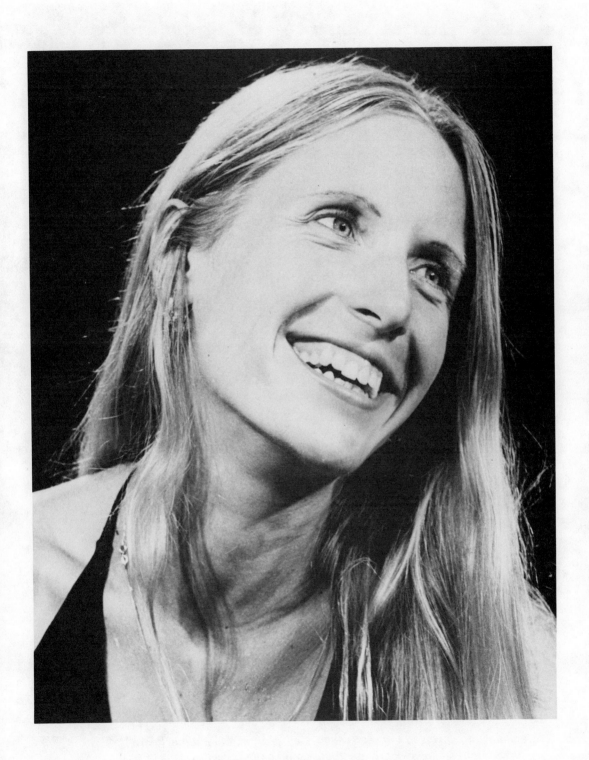

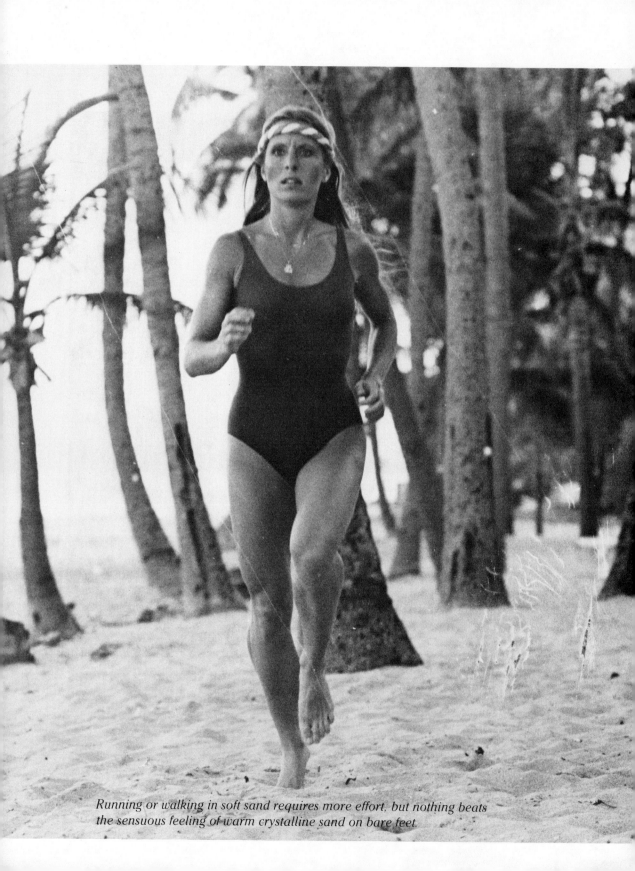

*Running or walking in soft sand requires more effort, but nothing beats the sensuous feeling of warm crystalline sand on bare feet.*

increase the intensity of these sprints until you can do fifteen at 95 percent of your maximum speed. Then increase the distance. (Save that last 5 percent for the Olympics.)

**Q.** When I'm sleeping, I'll often be rolling over in bed and stretching my legs, when suddenly I get a cramp in my leg that absolutely jolts me out of bed. What causes this?

**A.** Lack of certain nutrients in the surrounding tissue and bloodstream can force a muscle to contract involuntarily. Another type of cramp known as intermittent claudication is usually caused by build-up of fatty deposits in the arteries of the leg (atherosclerosis). This causes reduced blood supply to the extremities, resulting in chronic oxygen deficiency. Cramping and pain may occur whenever any type of exercise requiring more oxygen is performed, but unless you are diabetic, a smoker, or have cardiovascular disease, you are probably not in this category.

Pregnant or menstruating women, or women on the pill, often have leg pains which are generally related to higher estrogen levels, which create increased needs for vitamin E. Calcium needs are usually increased as well.

*Prevention of leg cramps:* Calcium and magnesium are very important minerals for muscle fiber relaxation. Calcium in our modern diet is usually low because high amounts of phosphorus tend to neutralize the calcium. Vitamin D is also required for calcium absorption—you get it free from sunlight or from fish liver oils. Many green vegetables, almonds, sesame seeds, comfrey, and yogurt are good calcium sources.

Increase of vitamins E, C, D, and the B complex, as well as supplemental calcium and magnesium are recommended by most experts.

If the "cramp phantom" strikes in the night, massage, gentle stretching, and warm compresses can alleviate the immediate pain. But *do* investigate preventive measures, and then sleep well.

**Q.** I've just started exercising, and my leg muscles must be really unused to it all, because they are very sore. Is there anything I can do for this until I get into better shape?

**A.** You may not want to hear this, but even *my* legs get sore after an especially hard workout—even when I'm in the best of condition.

Any time the muscle is worked to the point where the muscle glycogen (fuel) is depleted, then the muscle accumulates a waste by-product of the exertion: lactic acid. This is the main cause of muscle soreness from overwork.

Naturally, the more fit you become, the more work load the muscles can take before this overload occurs.

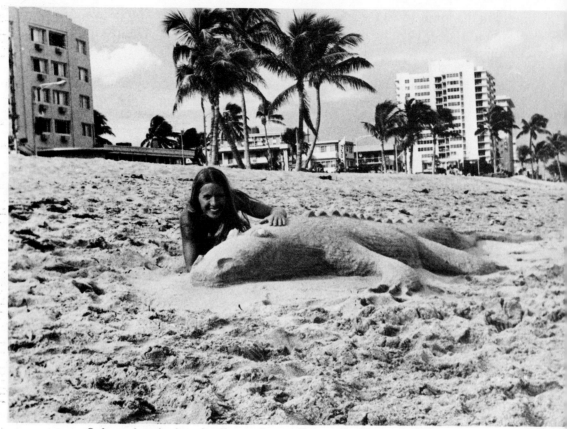

*Soft sand at the beach offers a demanding workout, but afterward a chance to have fun. On a Florida beach with a friend*

However, in the meantime, you may try increasing your intake of complex carbohydrates—whole grains, for instance, rice, bulgur, millet, baked potatoes, etc. I've found this to help me. In addition, be sure to increase your fluid intake to ensure proper hydration of the body. Eating a whole fresh pineapple also helps to restore the muscles by virtue of a proteolytic enzyme which eats away at dead tissue. Best of all the remedies for sore muscles, I've always found the most gratifying to be a long soak in a hot tub scented with sweet herbs.

**Q.** What are "shin splints" and how do you get rid of them?

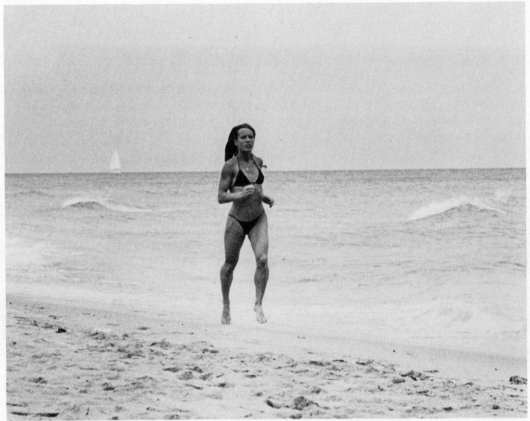

*Running by the ocean—footloose and fancy-free*

**A.** Shin splints is the lay term for tendinitis, which is inflammation or tearing of the tissue between the posterior and anterior tibialis muscle and the tibia. Most usual causes are poorly padded shoes, running on hard surfaces such as concrete, and immobility of the lower back, which causes weight-bearing through the leg to be executed at an unnatural and sometimes painful angle, as you have found.

Prevention: running on natural surfaces such as grass or dirt with an excellent pair of running shoes. You may also want to get your back checked out by a chiropractor to eliminate the possibility of a back problem.

What to do right now? Ice is the usual course of action. Rub the shins with an ice cube for about 10 minutes after you exercise. Of course, if pain persists, consult your podiatrist or family physician.

**Q.** Is there a way to tell if the workout was hard other than just by the way you feel?

**A.** After I run, row, swim, or cycle—and that's immediately upon stopping—I take my heart rate (put your fingertips directly over your heart to feel it, or under your jawbone halfway between your chin and your ear), counting one full minute. This shows two things:

**1.** If the 10-second count for me is 32 beats, then I know I have worked to my maximum heart rate. The American Heart Association says to find your rough maximum, take the number 220 and subtract your age. To figure out what this would be for 10 seconds, I divide by 6.

For instance, 220 minus 28 (my age) equals 192. To find out if my heart beats at that rate for those first 10 seconds—I'm counting after the workout—I divide by 6 (10 seconds being $\frac{1}{6}$ of a minute). That gives me $192 \div 6 = 32$. So a heart rate of 32 after my workout for the 10 count means I worked very hard.

**2.** Counting for the full minute tells more of a story. If my heart beat drops to under 100 beats for the whole minute, then it shows that my body was able to recover very quickly, and the workout was not that taxing. If my heart rate slows very little in that one minute after stopping the workout (say it's 160 beats for the full 60 seconds), then I know that not only did I work near my maximum heart rate (as the first 10 seconds told me) but my heart is not recovering quickly, so the next workout should be an easy one.

If you'd like to learn more about this kind of thing, then I strongly suggest Kenneth Cooper's book, *Aerobics* (New York City: Bantam, 1970).

P.S. And if you don't feel any pulse at all, get ready to sing the "Hallelujah Chorus"—you've made it!

**Q.** My sneakers really stink! I hate to throw them out, though. I paid $59.00 for them and they're hardly even worn out. Is there any way to get the smell out?

**A.** Your sneakers are suffering from a malady I call smell-o-vision! That is, you can smell 'em before you can see 'em. The answer: Throw them in the washing machine with some strong detergent. You can't wear them the way they are, so if they shrink, it's a risk you're willing to take, right? And if you use a cold water setting, they probably won't shrink. Then remove and throw away the insoles. Dry the shoes in the sun, stuffing newspaper in them to help them keep their form. Put in new insoles and wear socks with your shoes from now on. Keeping your sneakers just for

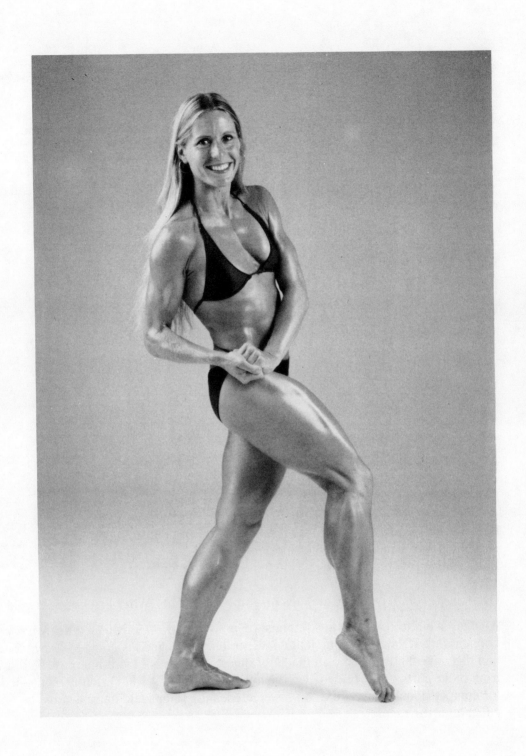

exercising allows them to dry out properly between sessions and prevents smell-o-vision. And if all this doesn't work, you can always hang them up and plant flowers in them.

**Q.** What's the big deal with vitamins? Certainly there's always a variety of food available in this country—how can you miss?

**A.** Read these charts and see how easily essential vitamins and minerals can be depleted. The following is a list of some of the more common elements that can deplete the body of vitamins:

| *Element* | *Vitamin* |
|---|---|
| Alcohol | B & C |
| Aspirin | C |
| Barbiturates | B |
| Caffeine | B, C |
| Chlorine dioxide (a bread preservative) | E |
| Light | $B_2$ |
| Rancid fat | E |
| Smoking | C (25 mg per cigarette) |
| Stress | B, C, A |

Some of the major minerals are depleted as follows:

| | |
|---|---|
| Absence of fruit and vegetables, table salt, caffeine, boiling food, stress, diuretics | Potassium |
| Caffeine, oxalic acid | Iron |
| Alcohol, chemically fertilized food | Magnesium |
| Caffeine, imbalance of protein, table salt, refined carbohydrates, pasteurized milk, fluoride | Calcium |
| Boiling food, refining of food | Trace minerals |

**Q.** Honey is often eaten by athletes prior to their events. Why? Is it good for you?

**A.** Bees seem to thrive on it, so it must be pretty good—giving us a quick energy boost, right? Wrong. Anything that concentrated and refined is going to draw blood and digestive fluids into the stomach for digestion. This is blood that must be drawn from other parts of the body—like the muscles—where it will certainly be needed for competition. Performance can be affected, and cramps and nausea could be an effect after the race.

Also, in sensitive individuals, a reactive hypoglycemia could be the result of a spoonful of honey at any time, not just before a race when your adrenaline is pumping. I took a swig of maple syrup once just before getting on the starting line in a 400-meter race. There were a couple of false starts, and after ten minutes of delays, I would have given a thousand dollars just to lie down and go to sleep right there on the track. The concentrated sweetness of the syrup had just the opposite effect I'd hoped for—I was literally drugged by it. The other lesson here is not to try out things on race day that you've never tried out before in workouts. The first lesson, of course, is that even though hummingbirds and bees might do it, it doesn't mean that it'll work for athletes.

**Q.** What is so terrible about frying food?

**A.** If you use an unsaturated fat, vitamin E is lost, and prolonged frying may turn the fat rancid. Think of restaurants that use the same fat for weeks at a time in preparing French fries, for instance, and you get the picture. Also, when frying with saturated fat, burning of the fat produces acrolein, a poison. Unnecessary calories are also added to the food by frying.

**Q.** I'm confused—the magazine commercials claim that their products are polyunsaturated fat. What's the difference between that and saturated fat? Is there unsaturated fat, too? And is one of them better than the others?

**A.** In a saturated fat, each carbon atom in the long chain molecule carries all of the hydrogen atoms possible. These fats are usually solid at room temperature, e.g., butter, lard, coconut oil.

Unsaturated fats are those in which one or more of the carbon atoms fails to carry all of the hydrogen atoms possible, and are usually liquid at room temperature, e.g., olive oil.

Polyunsaturated fats have more than one double bond in their molecular structure, and are found in fish, seed oils, and other softer foods.

For the record, there are also mono-unsaturated fats, having only one double bond and common in both plant and animal fats.

Your body uses fats for energy and warmth. Most nutrition authorities agree that a healthy diet should include more unsaturated fats than the others. The reason? These fats contain factors called "essential fatty acids" that the body needs to synthesize vitamins A, D, and E. However, each type of fat is needed by the body in some degree.

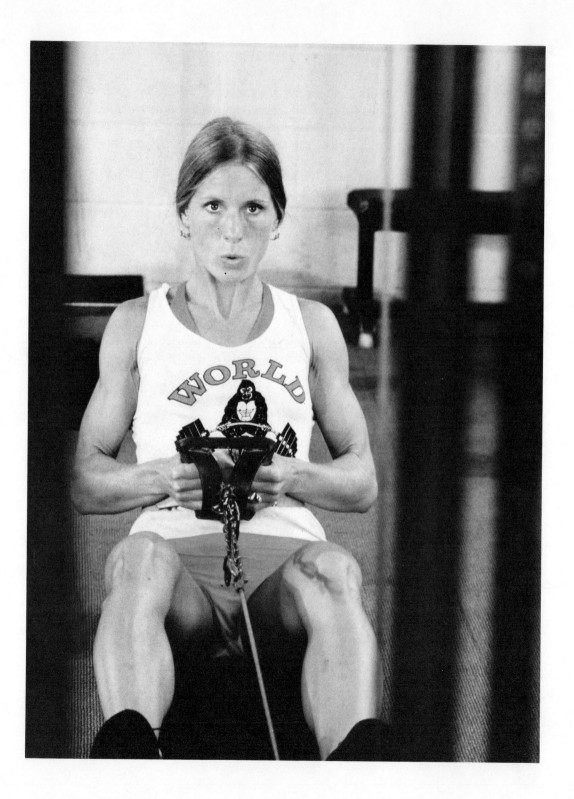

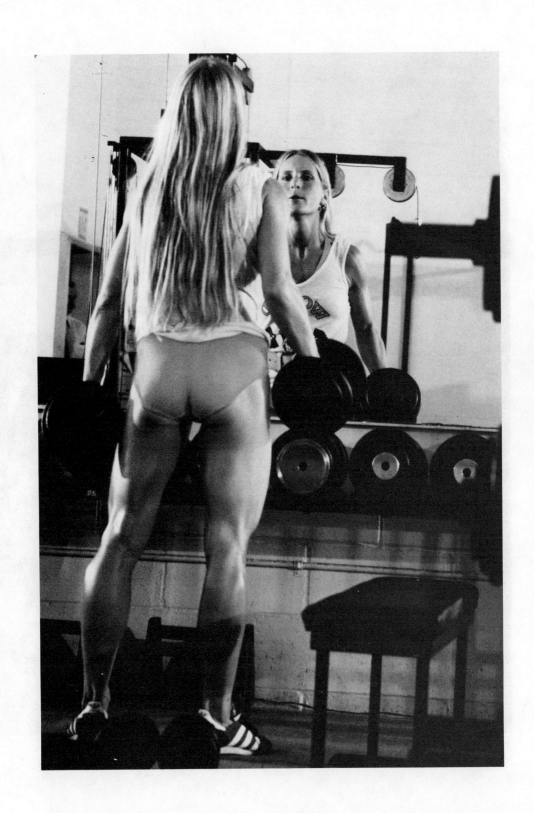

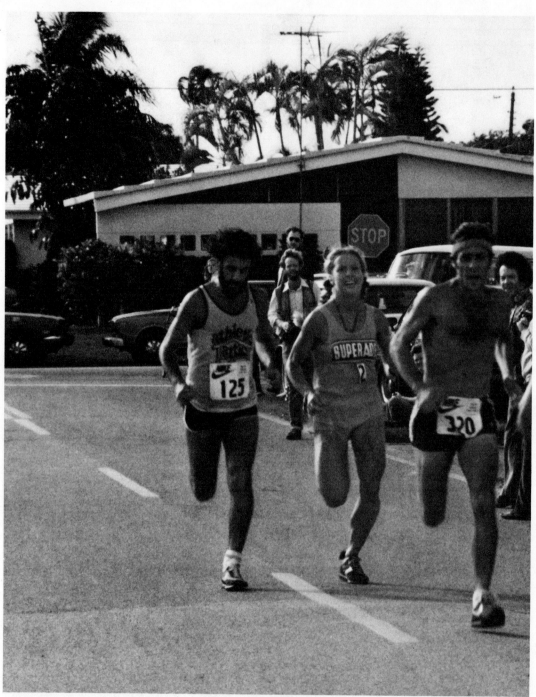

*Three-legged race!*

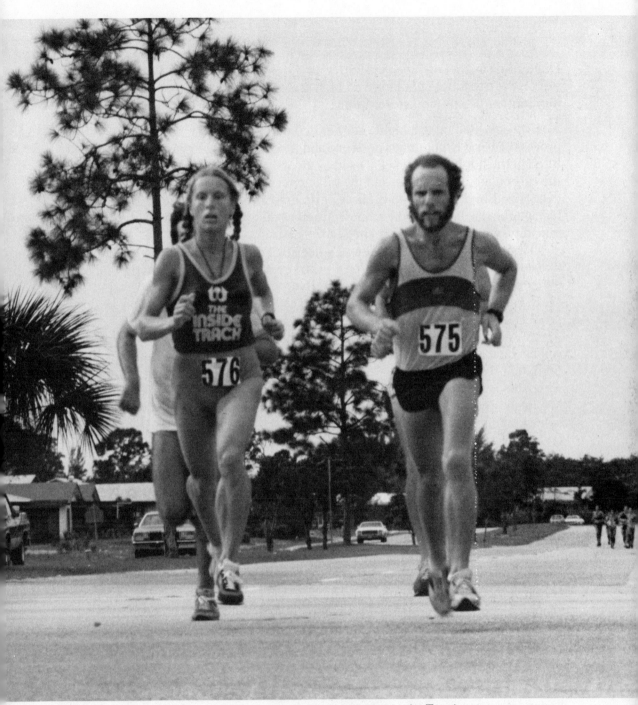

*A hot pace in a hot-weather race in the Tropics*

**Q.** Reading a label on a peanut-butter jar, I noticed that it said "No hydrogenated oil" on the front. But I could see an inch of oil floating on the top of the jar. Is this just another health-food store rip-off?

**A.** Hydrogenated oil is a highly adulterated oil that has gone through the following process: The oil is put under pressure and heated. Hydrogen gas is then bubbled through the hot liquid (nickel is used as a catalyst). The hydrogen combines with the carbon atoms in the oil, and the oil becomes solid. It is then bleached, deodorized, and filtered. Molecularly, it no longer resembles the original oil. It is highly artificial, but from the manufacturer's side, it vastly decreases the chance for rancidity, which means longer shelf life.

   From the body's point of view, it's like sticking the wrong key in the lock when it meets with hydrogenated fat. The wrong key doesn't work, but the right one won't either until you take the wrong one out. Hydrogenated fats act as anti-essential fatty acids. Lack of essential fatty acids is linked to cataracts, heart disease, and skin problems.

   Now, back to the peanut-butter jar. Peanut oil is usually hydrogenated so that it will become solid at room temperature. The oil separation you saw in the jar is proof that the label was true—the oil was unhydrogenated or simply untampered with. This is the better kind of peanut butter. Just buy it from a supplier who deals in a fresh product and stir it up when you get home. The best peanut butter, though, is the kind they make for you while you wait—fresh peanuts, skin and all, get ground up before your eyes and then you watch it go into your own jar. My logic says anything else but that is a rip-off.

**Q.** Having learned all that, what is partially hydrogenated oil?

**A.** A product is either hydrogenated or it isn't. This type of labeling is done to alleviate public concern at the hydrogenated process discussed earlier. It's like being a little bit pregnant. No such thing.

**Q.** Do you ever wake up in the morning and feel ugly, fat, and completely out of shape, even if you felt great the day before?

**A.** Absolutely. I know the feeling well! I've looked in the mirror on quite a few Monday mornings and winced—and this is after running about 30 miles the day before.

   It's unbelievable how bad you can feel on these days—even the tiniest imperfection can make you want to wear a brown paper bag over your head all day.

   This is a sign of fatigue, and on these "I feel ugly days" I usually plan something fun for a workout—maybe jumping up and down on a trampoline, rowing in the ocean, or running somewhere scenic—like by the ocean, or on a pine-needle trail.

For my mental attitude, I schedule a movie or some live music. Buy yourself a new red toothbrush. If your budget allows, treat yourself to that new record album you've wanted, or how about getting a massage?

Whatever you do, don't mope around brooding about the fact that you feel less than perfect. If you're worrying about how you think people see you, remember that not everyone has 20-20 vision.

**Q.** Can you really spot-reduce with vibrator belts, sauna wraps, and rubber sweatsuits? My husband wears one of those thick rubber wraparounds and he swears by it, but frankly, I don't see any difference on him. At least at my spa, I figure that the vibrator belt will help me lose a few inches because it's a massage. We have a bet on this. Who is right?

**A.** You're both wrong. There's no such thing as spot reducing. Now you can firm up any area by exercise, but those sauna wraps and your husband's rubber wraparound only promote perspiration. The fat remains to haunt you. And those vibrator belts can do wonders for aching muscles, but the fat they jiggle only gets tickled, and it doesn't fall off you. I'm sorry you both lost the bet, but with the extra time on your hands because of this resolved predicament, take heart. That cloth-backed spongy rubber from your husband's wraparound is the very stuff used in the fanciest of insoles by the running elite. Cut out a pair for each other and have enough left over for a new pair on your birthdays!

**Q.** What about these machines that are supposed to exercise your muscles while you just lie there? Are they really any good? Are there side effects?

**A.** There *are* machines now that can cause the muscles to contract through electric current. Here's how it works:

Rubber or plastic electrodes are placed on the skin along with an electroconductive gel or water. These electrodes are generally placed on the muscle and then mild electrical current is turned on. You feel the muscle contracted and relaxed involuntarily.

Depending on how strong the current is, and how long the electrodes are left on one spot, there is a toning of the muscles involved. There are salons around the country that will give you a half-hour session with a dozen or more electrodes on different muscles. One side effect could be lactic acid, if the electrical current is too strong, and sore muscles will be the result, just as if you overworked the muscles in the usual way.

This whole concept has been around for years, but is just now being commercialized. Previously it was used mainly as an aid in physical therapy.

However, getting the muscles worked by a machine is really just a prop for those who want fitness without effort. The effect of the machines on developing a strong and healthy heart is marginal.

If you are still curious to try this out for yourself, *do* look for trained personnel in the salon you visit. If the staff's credentials are not visibly displayed, walk out. Naturally, your Better Business Bureau is always a way to check out the place further, if you have any doubts.

A few parting thoughts—these machines *do* have a toning effect on the muscles, but for total fitness you still must make your heart beat faster every day— on your own. And besides, *getting* there on your own steam is more than half the fun.

# EPILOGUE

Depending on your eagerness to improve, and how demanding you've been on yourself, these last six weeks will have changed you.

Now you should be able to see differences in your clothes—they will fit you differently. Your measurements alone will tell part of the story—another part will be told by your own reflection in the mirror.

But the most important thing is that you have begun to take care of yourself. You've shown *yourself* in the past six weeks that you are a person who succeeds in your fitness program. This will carry over into other parts of your life. When you have a lithe and active body, it is a source of pleasure to you, and the harmony it brings shines through your whole person.

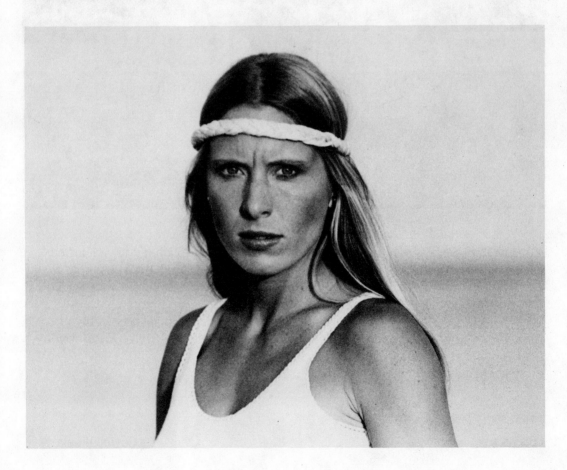

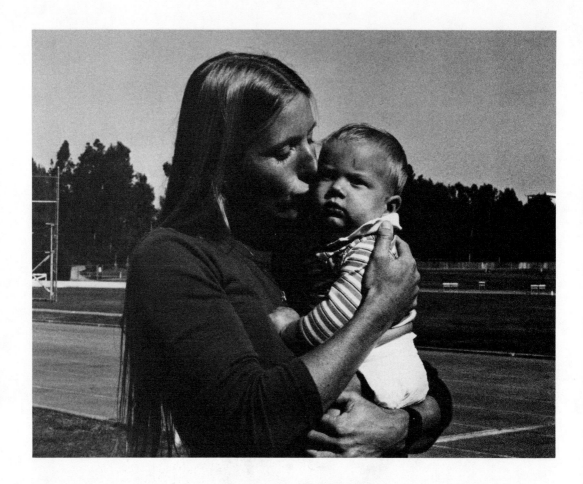

Invent new ways to stay in shape now, and add them to what you've learned already. And be sure to keep a sharp and critical eye on your figure—a simple record of your measurements every month keeps you accountable to yourself, so that you can keep on looking great forever!

Thank you for allowing me to share some of my shape-up secrets with you. Have you discovered that strength is beautiful? Because that's what I wish for you— the beauty of your own strength, always.

Stay healthy and enjoy your super legs.

Gayle Olinekova

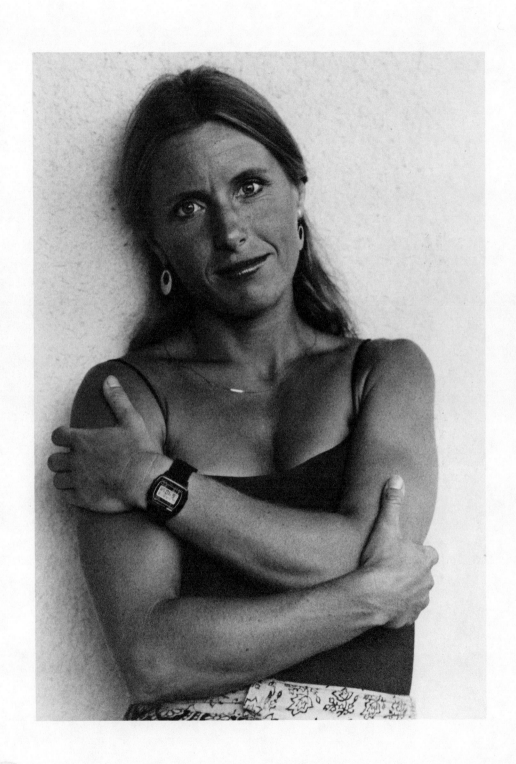